DEATH DYING & DONUTS

Dr Colin Dicks

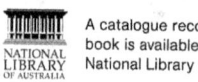 A catalogue record for this book is available from the National Library of Australia

Death, Dying & Donuts
Copyright 2022 ©Dr Colin Dicks

Published by Star Label Publishing
P.O. Box 1511, Buderim, QLD, Australia
publishing@starlabel.com.au

Editing: David Goodwin, Mandy Chandler, Katie Lawry
Interior design and editing: Rebecca Moore
Cover art: Andre Eberle

1st Edition November, 2022
All rights reserved. No part of this publication may be reproduced in any form; stored in a retrieval system; or transmitted; or used in any other form; or by any other means without prior written permission of the publisher (except for brief quotes for the purpose of review or promotion).

The views expressed here-in remain the sole responsibility of the author, who exempts the publisher from all liability. The author and publisher do not assume responsibility for any loss, damage, or disruption caused by the contents, errors or omissions, whether such contents, errors, or omissions result from opinion, negligence, accident, or any other cause, and hereby disclaim any and all liability to any party.

ISBN: 978-0-6453697-2-4

Endorsements

Even as a physician of 50 years' standing, I found I was woefully unprepared to cope with the short illness and death of my wife. Colin allowed me to review the manuscript during the last days of my wife's illness, and I found it immensely helpful. This book will enable the dying and the soon-to-be-bereaved to face the reality of dying with humanity. We can aspire to a "good death" for our loved ones and ourselves.

Dr John Clements AM

Dr Colin offers a unique perspective on an experience we all must face. Sensitive, yet intensely practical; beautifully kind, yet directly addressing the fears we all have; this book is essential reading for both carers and those dying.

It is written by a man who walks this road every day, and hence is uniquely qualified to equip every person for their personal journey into death. I recommend this to every person facing death that I know, and the knowledge Colin shares brings great comfort and direction to all who are preparing to face death.

Pastor Darin Browne

Death, Dying & Donuts is essential reading to prepare yourself for the full journey of life from birth to death...and helped me understand much more clearly the journey that my ageing parents are travelling, thank you Colin.

Larissa Meyer

With years of experience, deep empathy and a gentle sense of humour Dr Dicks takes you by the hand and guides you on the difficult path of death and dying.

Whether it is for you, or somebody close to you, this book enables you to navigate the unfamiliar terrain that comes with death and dying emotionally, spiritually, physically and practically.

With Dr Dicks accompanying you every step along the way, *Death, Dying and Donuts* is an essential resource that shouldn't be missed.

Anna-Marie Lombard

Are you or a loved one faced with the reality of death and dying? Finding yourself asking questions such as, "Why me? What is true? Where do I come from? Where will I go? What is valuable to me?

In my professional opinion, as a counsellor and psychotherapist and with my personal experience as a daughter who lost her mother to cancer at a young age, I can highly recommend this book to everyone who is confronted with the existential questions surrounding death and dying.

This book will not only give you the confidence to talk about an inevitable and challenging topic namely death, but it will also help you understand the normal challenges faced and even make it a more bearable process.

Furthermore, it may help anyone in their search for the meaning of such suffering when faced with difficult choices. Victor Franklyn wrote in his book *Man's Search for Meaning*, "Once an individual's search for a meaning is successful, it not only renders him happy but also gives him the capability to cope with suffering" (p.14).

I do believe this book was inspired and am grateful that Colin Dicks rose to this challenge when he wrote this book as I believe it will help many others.

Henrietta Oosthuizen
Counsellor, Family Therapist,
Psychotherapist, Supervisor, Trainer, and Assessor.

Table of Contents

Foreword ix

Preface xi

1. Introduction to Death & Dying 1

2. Death's Reputation 7

3. The Character of Death 15

4. The Iceberg Moment 23

5. The Changing Narrative 31

6. The Death Code, Ageing & Why We Die 41

7. Physical Death 47

8. Physical Aspects of Dying 55

9. Introduction To Emotions 65

10. Fear, Anxiety & Worry 79

11. Loss & Grief 87

12. Anger 95

13. Depression & Sadness In Loss..101

14. Guilt & Regret...107

15. Emotional Responsibility..115

16. Faith & Hope...123

17. Introduction To Spirituality...131

18. Near Death Experiences...137

19. Spiritual Awakening...143

20. Exposure To God..149

21. Into The Storm..157

22. Action Stations...169

23. Communicating Legal & Financial Matters..........................177

24. Funeral Planning..185

25. Make Provision For Illness & Death.......................................193

26. Palliative Care Heroes..201

27. The Unsung Heroes...207

28. Bereavement..213

29. Looking The Other Way & Donuts...........................217

30. Putting It All Together..225

31. Dying To Understand...229

Epilogue...231

About The Author..234

FOREWORD

As a colleague of Dr Colin Dicks for many years within the oncology field, I am privileged to write the foreword for this important piece of work.

I approached the reading of Colin's new book from two perspectives. The first was as a colleague of Colin's, having worked with him in the past and valuing his perspective and help in the treatment of patients with terminal diseases, who were in need of symptom relief. The second was as a medical oncologist and palliative care physician with over 60 years' experience of treating patients with terminal disease who were going through the dying process.

Therefore, I was surprised to find myself reading it more as an older individual contemplating the dying process itself from my own perspective more than I did that of the impartial observer that I have been for many years.

I found Colin's writing very thoughtful and, in places, quite humorous. I feel I need to go back and re-read many parts of the book and take the quotes and anecdotes as things that I could use with my patients, or to make them part of my experience for the final test to come. As somebody who knows the strong spiritual side that

Colin has, I wondered if this would intrude into the book somehow. I was pleasantly surprised to discover that this was not the case. I do, however, highly recommend you read his story in the epilogue. It is one that could easily be ignored if you felt inclined to do so, but I believe that it is worthwhile to look at his approach and see if it does actually contain something that might be useful and helpful for you during this journey. I believe it is beneficial to consider all possibilities while you are still able.

I would like to give this book to all my family members, as well as friends and patients, because I believe it contains many nuggets of truth that will help all of us in this journey that, as Colin says, is a test nobody wants to take, but we all must. As Colin states, we can, however, be assured that nobody has ever failed.

I hope that this book becomes widely read and required reading for all hospice and palliative care workers as well as their patients. I look forward to the TED talks and interviews.

Dr Geoffrey A T Hawson

MBBS FRACP FAChPM Dip. Clin Hyp. FRCPA (1976)
Associate Professor (UQ)
Haematologist Oncologist

PREFACE

As a radiation oncologist, I use radiation to cure cancer. While this may seem a noble ambition, not all cancers can be cured. The other, less pleasant part of my job is the difficult conversation when a cure is not possible. Here, death is the endgame, and these conversations are often awkward.

No one wants to talk about death and dying—we prefer to pretend that we don't have to die; we prefer to ignore this huge problem.

Yet death is the one thing we all have in common—it is the one thing that unites us all. It is the one thing that is absolutely certain and unavoidable. It is our destiny to die and, because of this, it is astonishingly irresponsible not to know anything about death or to prepare for dying.

We are not usually this negligent with other things in life. We routinely prepare for future events. We prepare for holidays, exams or weddings because we want the best outcomes when these events take place. We want to enjoy our holiday or pass the exam, and when it comes to a wedding, we like to make sure everything is perfect. But it seems that when it comes to dying, which is arguably one of the most important things we get to do in life, we are often content to hope for the best and leave it to chance.

Why is this so?

It is because of ignorance. We fear that which we do not understand. The purpose of this book is to shed light on this thing called 'death' and to make it acceptable. Some may object and argue that, "Death will never be acceptable!" or "I plan to live forever." These are noble thoughts, but they are not wise thoughts. They are our enemy when it comes to having a good death. Wishful thinking is exactly that—wishful! We need more than this when it comes to dying.

In 2014, I wrote and self-published *About dying: how to live in the face of death* to start a conversation about dying and normalise death. The feedback I received was encouraging, and as much as the book was a start, it was not enough.

In 2019, I undertook research to discover what people knew about dying. I asked what death education was being offered to people with terminal cancer. I thought of education as you would think of coaching—I wanted to know what coaching or skills people were given to empower them to meet the challenges of dying. The shocking response from the majority of people to the research question was a resounding, "NONE!"

Although those dying were well supported by the medical team with sufficient medical appointments, good care and well wishes, they knew next to nothing about dying. This knowledge remained the secret of the healthcare professionals. Those affected by dying remained ignorant about what lay ahead, and this ignorance came at a great cost.

It cost them time, and time is one thing you don't have when you are dying. They spent time fighting death when they could have been spending time doing what they loved. They did not understand the changes happening in their body or the symptoms they could expect when life was ending. They did not fully understand the wild emotions at play when life is ending, and for some, the spiritual issues around dying were illuminating.

There were many things they knew they had to do, but the detail of these were often lost in the chaos of illness, medical appointments and the emotions associated with dying. Because they did not know what to expect or to do, people made mistakes; they made the wrong choices, and they often ended up feeling abandoned and without hope.

The other thing I learnt was that people do not die in isolation. Death affects all those on the journey—not only the person dying. This was the most startling discovery from my research—that dying is a team effort, and that the patient and the carer are both caught up in the process of dying, each in their own unique way. Both experience loss and feel the pain of dying but in different ways. Those caring for the dying often feel forgotten or neglected.

There was a cry for a user-friendly resource on dying by those in the research group who had been through bereavement. This is my honest attempt at providing this resource. It is based on my observations as an oncologist, my experience of bereavement, my view of spirituality, and my desire to provide a roadmap for the end of life.

This map will not provide all the answers. There may be things that you do not agree with, and there may be points of view that are stumbling blocks. Please don't let that deter you. I suggest that you skip the parts you don't like. There is something in here for everyone: for those dying, for the carers and families of those dying, and for health professionals who need a way to say, "Let's have this conversation about dying."

When it comes to dying, there are no professionals. We all get to die once, and although we cannot rely on personal past experiences to equip us for our death, we can observe the experiences of others. I do not know all the answers, so please share your experiences with me at admin@dyingtounderstand.com so that together, we can all keep learning. I am not providing professional advice, so please talk to your own doctor and support team about this.

As I am not dying (yet), please forgive me for any insensitivity or lack of insight. This is not an academic reference book. The examples I use in the book are about real people. To protect their identities, I have changed their names and their stories without losing the meaning of their experience.

I do not work with children and the issue of children dying is not addressed in this book. Though I cannot imagine the pain a parent feels when their child dies, I know that finding professional help through the grief and loss is important. I believe that children are far more resilient than we give them credit for, and that honesty is an important part of the conversation with children. They have an inherent faith and if there is a hope of going home to God, they will be comforted and ready (Matthew 18:10).

When it comes to dying, there are important physical, emotional, spiritual and practical things to consider. There is no denying that dying is difficult. It is associated with loss and suffering, and those left behind must endure the winter of bereavement. This is the nature of death, but it is only part of the story. There is more to death than just loss and suffering.

This book is not only about dying, it is also an invitation to get on with living. While death and dying are not negotiable, how we choose to live is. Even in the face of death, we can do the things that we like doing. Some people like painting, others like playing music, bushwalking, or going on a cruise. I like eating donuts. For me, there's something very satisfying about sinking my teeth through the sugary cinnamon outside, then into the sweet fluffy dough beneath. Add a coffee and I have perfect happiness. Though it lasts only for a short time, it's enjoyable and I know that tomorrow there could be another one to enjoy. These small, seemingly insignificant things can add moments of happiness to a day that may otherwise seem grey, and these moments matter.

Whether you enjoy a good donut like me, or whatever your pleasure, the point of life is that we enjoy it, and make the most of it while we are alive. We have the opportunity to make our lives count and, when life is ending, perhaps count even more. This is where we may find that even little things can make a big difference to a day.

If we let the fear of death get in the way of enjoying life, we miss out. If we dare to change our thinking about dying, we may be convinced that death is not as bad as we may have imagined. And for those who choose to believe, there is the assurance that death is not the end of the road, but rather the doorway to the next great adventure.

So, grab yourself a donut and settle in while we explore this confronting, yet inevitable stage of life.

Chapter 1

Introduction to Death & Dying

As a young doctor, I had two dying patients under my care. One patient, Mrs Blades, was at peace about this. She accepted that her time had come. She and her husband chuckled away about things, held hands, and demonstrated their love for each other. In the sadness of her approaching death, they were both happy and content. They accepted death as a part of life, and there was no struggle against this approaching certainty. I would visit her room and spend time chatting with them; there was not much else we could do. I used to look forward to these visits because she always left me feeling valued, and on the day her room was empty, I felt the loss. But it was a loss without a sting; it was a happy kind of loss, with hope and thankfulness for having been able to care for her and share a small part of her life. I think she had a good death.

I was also caring for Frances at the same time. Her last days were a battle to stay alive. She fought death, and every day the battle was intense. Though she did her best, ultimately, she lost. Her death was in stark contrast to that of Mrs Blades. Frances was not ready to die, and in her dying, there was a different kind of loss—one of defeat, sadness and fear. She did not have an easy death.

There can never be a truly easy death, but it may be possible to have a good death. This won't happen by wishful thinking—it requires different thinking. It requires a deliberate approach to put 'death' and 'good' next to each other and allow them to coexist. It requires a willingness to understand death and, where possible, to make peace with death. But how do we make peace with death if it is there to destroy us?

Well, that will depend on what we mean by 'us'. This is at the heart of the matter: the concept of being, of who we are and what we are here for. It will depend on what we mean by death and what we mean by life. Without a clear understanding of these concepts, we may be fooled into believing that death is always evil and to be avoided at all costs.

The concept of 'self' is the most difficult one to consider. It is perhaps best demonstrated by asking the question, "Who are you?" I would answer, "Colin Dicks" but that is just my name, it does not tell you about who I am. To understand who I am would require an understanding about my values and beliefs, likes and dislikes, character, relationships, achievements and failures, roles and responsibilities, and my culture and family context.

While death may be able to destroy my physical body, it is unable to delete the story of my life, my values, my beliefs, or my character. It may end my future relationships and friendships, but it cannot take away the depth, colour and joy of all the relationships and friendships I have lived through and enjoyed. It may prevent me participating in life, but it cannot take away what I have achieved and accomplished in life. It cannot eliminate the role I have in my family. I will always be my children's father and my wife's husband. All that I am remains after I am no longer here. My life cannot be undone.

As mortals, we have a finite period of time on Earth. Death is not evil, it is merely the evidence that we have run out of time. Sometimes by misfortune this time is far shorter than we expected, and this is unfair. Sometimes this time is longer than we wanted, and this is also unfair.

When James was diagnosed with dementia, it did not seem to be too bad. It was manageable, but it became unmanageable when he lost his way at the end of life. All that he was, his achievements, character, friendships and values, were threatened by the 'new' person he had become due to his illness. Death could not come soon enough. He went into 'overtime' and for those who work with dementia or care for someone with dementia, this is a tragedy.

If death is 'running out of time' then life must be how we use our time. There are those who are living but they are not alive. They exist, but they do not make use of their time. They fail to explore, enjoy or experience life. They miss out on this wonderful gift of life that is offered to each of us every day. They misdirect their time to pursue unimportant matters.

In my work, I often see people who paradoxically benefit from a life-threatening cancer diagnosis. They come to understand that time is valuable and not to be wasted, and they redirect their lives to make the most of their remaining time. They invest in things of permanent value, such as experiences, memories and friendships. They willingly relinquish their place at the board meeting so that they can have more quality time and do those things that matter more often. Things like the pleasure of gardening, walking on the beach, or feeling the golden warmth of sunshine. Even the little things that give us pleasure matter. We owe it to ourselves to enjoy some of our time, even if it is in a small and trivial way every day.

That's why we need donuts. As I mentioned in the preface, I like eating donuts. For me, biting into the soft doughiness of a cinnamon-and-sugar-coated donut is a good feeling. Add coffee to the equation and my happiness is complete. I don't need donuts every day, but on a good day—why not? And on a bad day—why not even more? It is not always the big things, but rather the small and everyday things that we enjoy that matter, and declare, "We are alive!" While we have time, it is our responsibility to use the time and to enjoy it because, before we know it, our time might be running out.

We may identify this period when we run out of time as the period when we are dying. This is a time of enormous transition where we go from perfect health to no health at all. For some, this happens in an instant and they are unable to say goodbye or tidy up the loose ends in their life. These deaths are tragic and leave those who are left behind with the deepest wounds.

I think the fortunate ones are those who have a small period to prepare for death when life is ending. They have an opportunity to die like Mrs Blades, packed and ready to go, leaving behind a good life with no regrets. They can have a good death.

This book is not about dying today, but about being prepared for death for some day in the future. May you be blessed with a long life, and may you, in whatever time you have left, have the opportunity to live every day as if it were your last one.

But, for that last day, there is work to be done. To have a good death, we need to understand what is at stake. We need to know the rules of the game. We need to know about death if we want to win.

Chapter 2

Death's Reputation

Death has a bad reputation, and it is not always death's fault. If death were to object to the slander and take its case to a court, it would certainly win. We have a very negative view about dying, but this is mostly our fault. We have believed our own propaganda, and this has been to our disadvantage. We have created our own nightmare by saying that death is the worst thing that is ever going to happen, only to watch and see that we all eventually have to die. What a cruel prank.

If we are ever going to be able to face death, we have to start by facing the lies we have believed. Simply saying death sucks and then walking away from the topic is being unfair to ourselves because we have a future appointment with death. If anything, we owe it to ourselves to have a strategy when it comes to dying.

Our misunderstanding is based on the following factors:

Death's reputation

If you listen to the language around death, you will hear words like 'terrible', 'tragic' and 'awful', and the list goes on. Words are powerful and they convey powerful messages. Advertising copywriters know this and use words to create emotion out of language. For example, a simple word from a car dealer could sway you away from buying a Ford. Perhaps something such as 'unsafe'? Or, if someone told you that the ice-cream you just bought tastes like urine, chances are that you won't enjoy it as much as you did only a few seconds ago.

When it comes to death, we only hear negative language and words that convey fear and loss. These words are repeated in TV shows and dramas where death is made out to be the ultimate failure, the worst thing that can possibly happen, and the end of the world.

Added to this is the human tendency to embellish a story. What may have started off as a reasonably boring everyday death becomes a horror movie scene in the hands of the right person. Instead of old Aunt Agatha dying peacefully in her sleep, it becomes a graphic description of how her eyes popped out and her tongue was swollen when she died and how terrible it all was. But, if you'd cared to ask, her eyes popped out all her life and she always had a swollen tongue. Death had nothing to do with the fact that poor Aunt Agatha was quite ugly—but why waste a good story?

If we keep telling ourselves that death is terrible, we will come to believe it after a while. It will seem impossible to consider that someone could die happily or that they could die in peace. It is time to turn our language about death away from words that create fear and terror. Better words about death are 'normal', 'everyday', and 'expected'.

Uncertainty about death

No one really knows what happens when we die. We assume it to be a terrible thing, but is it really? The experience of death is usually from the point of view of those who have been left behind and they are reporting death from a perspective of loss and bereavement. No wonder death seems so terrible.

Some of those who have died and returned to tell the story of their near-death experiences (NDEs) no longer fear death. Paradoxically, if given the choice, they often say that they would prefer not to be here, and they long to return to their experience of heaven. From their spiritual vantage point, death is no longer a threat.

We tend to fear the unknown. It is easy to think that the fear we have of the unknown is our fear of death, but they are two different things. We can't be sure that death will be bad. If death is the release of physical suffering, it may even be good. For those with faith and an expectation of heaven, the last day on Earth may just turn out to be the best day.

Sanitisation of death

No one likes a mess and death can be messy. People die, and if we don't tidy it up, the streets would be littered with dead bodies. While this did happen at times in the past, thankfully, it does not happen today. People still die, but their bodies are not left unattended. As a society, we have not only learnt to dispose of the bodies, but we have also seemingly disposed of death.

These days, most of us never see death, but this was not the case a century ago. Back then, adults and children died of all sorts of everyday diseases, such as diphtheria and tuberculosis. In 1920, the average life expectancy was less than 55 years, and you would have been 'quite old' at the age of 60. If someone died, it was an everyday event and the body was kept at home on display, while preparations were made for the funeral. Relatives would come in and pay their respects. Death was a normal part of life.

Today, although death is as busy as ever, it's hard to find any evidence of it. When someone dies, they usually die in hospital, or if they die at home, the body is quickly removed. Even at the hospital the body is bathed, cleaned and covered up with a sheet. The ugliness of death is purified, and the now-not-so-offensive dead body is transported to the furthest reaches of the hospital—its morgue—where it remains hidden safely in a fridge.

When disposing of the body, traditional burials are less common, and more people are opting for cremation. Between the moment of death and the handful of ashes in an urn, there may be very little physical evidence that death has occurred. Today, when it comes to dying, it's not messy. "Nothing to see here, move right along."

When did you last see a dead body? Have you ever seen one? To modern eyes, a corpse is confronting, and if anyone saw a dead body today, they would probably be offered counselling. Why? Why have we made things so complicated? This abnormal response to death makes dying worse. In trying to protect ourselves from death, we have inevitably made it more terrifying.

Expectations and disappointment

We can trap ourselves by our expectations. If our expectations are realistic and important to us and we miss them, we will feel disappointment. Our disappointment is proportionate to our expectation: the greater the expectation, the greater the disappointment. If there is no expectation, there can be no disappointment.

I am not an athlete, so if I do not win a gold medal at the Olympics, I would not be disappointed because I have no expectation to ever win or even compete. In contrast, if an Olympic athlete won a silver medal, they may feel enormous disappointment despite their amazing achievement. This is because their expectation to win a gold medal was a realistic and important one. Winning a silver medal may be worse than winning a bronze medal because achieving silver meant they were so close to attaining gold!

These are realistic expectations for both me and an Olympic athlete. But what if I did feel devastated and disappointed and threw the furniture around because I had not won a gold medal, even though I did not compete? You would laugh at me and say, "That is unrealistic—you are being silly." If I feel disappointed by an unrealistic expectation, then the joke is on me.

But that is what happens when it comes to dying. If we have an unrealistic expectation to live forever and behave badly when this is not going to happen, the joke is on us. If, however, our expectation is realistic and we accept that we are all mortal, we will avoid disappointment when death visits.

We need to reset our expectations, especially in modern medicine, where we have the illusion that we can fix or cure anything. Even if we were to find the cure for all diseases, death would still pay us all a visit eventually. It is best to expect that knock on the door and be ready for it, rather than living life hoping that death will never come.

Accountability and assigning blame

We strive to live in a society where accountability is important. If something goes wrong, we feel it is essential to get to the root cause, to find out who or what was responsible, and then carry out remedial management so that we can avoid it happening again. This is a good practice when dealing with things that are under our control, but what about those that are not?

In 2011, the world's second most significant nuclear disaster occurred in the Fukushima Danchi Nuclear Reactor. The catastrophe was caused by the Tōhoku earthquake, which, at a magnitude of nine on the Richter Scale, was the fourth-most powerful earthquake ever recorded. It was so powerful, it shifted the Earth's axis by 10–25cm, causing a tsunami 14 metres high (more than four storeys) that swamped the reactor. At its peak, the wall of water would have been close to 40 metres high and travelling at 700 kilometres per hour.

An independent investigation concluded that Fukushima was a man-made disaster, and the energy company was blamed for failing to meet safety requirements or plan for such an event. But while it's easy to ask how this could happen, how do you plan for an event like that?

Finger pointing has become the norm in modern society. When something goes wrong, we seek to assign blame and it follows that if someone dies, someone must be at fault. Royal commissions and inquiries, hand wringing and soul searching all happens when there are deaths involved. But here's the newsflash: death is inevitable. And, just like the Fukushima disaster, there is nothing we can do about it.

That doesn't mean that we should be irresponsible. Things such as seat belts, airbags or bicycle helmets give us a better chance of surviving an accident, but we do need to get a grip and realise that, ultimately, we have no power over death. There is nothing we can do to prevent death.

It takes orders from no one. It is autonomous and arrives with or without notice. It is not concerned about good management skills, and it pays no attention to our demands that it should stay away.

Death simply happens. It is part of life. It does not sneak up on us and catch us unaware, it just does what it has always done. It has always been there, and it puts us on notice of its intention at birth. This life is finite—it will end, and every day we get to live before it does is a gift. We have been the deceitful ones by denying it is a normal part of life.

Death will mind its own business and we must as well. It will take care of itself. Our obligation is to get on with life.

We need to understand the place of death so that we can fully appreciate the gift of life.

Chapter 3

The Character of Death

Once we get the "ooh, death is so terrible" notion out of the way, it is possible to start looking at death objectively. Once we understand the nature of death, its terrifying mysteriousness is lost. It is then possible to start planning and devising strategies to cope with death so that it is no longer a threat to our enjoyment of life.

Have you ever considered the character of death? Death has commonly been personified in modern times as the Grim Reaper. In Greek mythology, death was personified as Thanos, a kindly old man who gathers the soul at the end of life. In East Asia, death dispensed justice in the afterlife as Yama. Death is one of the apocalyptical riders in the Bible's Book of Revelation. Throughout myth and legend, death is personified as a god-like being whose purpose is to harvest the souls of men and women. If we imagine death as an entity, visiting those whom he chooses at the time that he chooses, we can perhaps venture a look in his direction—hoping that he won't be looking back just yet.

We all probably know more about death than we think, it is just that we don't put aside the time to examine it as we should. Consider the following statements and see if you agree.

Death is a natural event
If you are a carbon-based lifeform, you are destined to die. While only a few animals have a lifespan of hundreds of years, most of us will do better than the poor old mayfly, which has a life expectancy of mere minutes. It lives, reproduces and dies in a blaze of glory. As humans we can expect to get around 70 years or so, but by the time we reach the century mark, our physical bodies are ready for recycling. If you don't believe me, ask a few nonagenarians their opinion on the subject—life at 90 is rarely fun.

Dying is normal
Statistically, dying is the most normal event ever, with a probability of 100%. Though the ways we die may vary, and some may be quite unique, the end result is the same—everyone ends up dead.

Death is unavoidable
Good health, fitness, yoga, medication, Pilates, diet, vitamins and superfoods are not going to prevent you from dying. While they may delay a premature death, they can't protect us forever. Nor can prayer, miracles, pilgrimages, magic or wishful thinking repel death. Being a health

fanatic may add a few extra miles on the journey of life, but the road eventually comes to an end for all.

We don't really mind death

It may come as a surprise, but most of us are generally unconcerned by death. We really don't care about the 150,000 people who die each day unless we are directly affected. The death rate in Brazil or the Congo doesn't bother us, unless we live there. We are often the instigators of death when it comes to vermin or roaches. There is nothing better than a dead roach.

Death is not biased

Death is no respecter of persons. Kings, queens, rulers, celebrities, the rich, the poor; all die in the same way. Wealth or titles or fame make no difference to death. Being super-famous just means others will know when you have died, it won't make you any less dead when your time comes. Death is impartial. It happened to Queen Elizabeth II, Michael Jackson, Diego Maradona and Sean Connery with the same finality as it happened to Joe, the guy who lived down the street, last night.

Death has no cargo space

We can't take anything with us when we die. The wealth and goods we accumulate in life are left behind, and the sum total of all the assets that we can take with us at the time of death is zero. We come into this world with nothing, and we leave this world with nothing. The ancient Egyptian pharaohs did everything they could to take their wealth with them into the afterlife, but they failed. Their treasure stayed for us to find—thank you for thinking of us, guys.

Death makes no exceptions and accepts no ransom
Everyone dies. There is no ransom you can pay to escape death. Even if you are cute, you aren't safe from death's calling card. It is not possible to bargain or charm your way out of it. Mastercards and Visa cards are always declined. It may be possible to buy the world, but no amount can 'pay off' death.

Death has its own timing
Death arrives at its own time. For some, it arrives at birth, way too soon to seem fair. For others, who have had enough of old age or suffering, it can't come soon enough. It controls its own timing, no one else does. I have always been struck by the extremes of the circumstances in which people die. One person may die after being stung by a little bee, yet another survives severe and extensive trauma that should have taken their life. Go figure!

Death is irreversible
Once dead always dead, there is no coming back for a second chance. There is no opportunity to tell people what you really meant in your will. You can't come back and say "I love you" or "I forgive you" when your time has passed.

This life is not a dress rehearsal. It is the real deal, the whole show, and it runs toward the one and only final curtain.

Death is painful
There is no escaping the pain of death. People fear the physical pain of death, but this is often less keenly felt than the emotional and sometimes spiritual pain experienced in dying. It is here that we touch on the exposed nerve that makes dying so unbearable. It is the pain we feel in grief, the pain we feel in saying goodbye. It hurts to die.

Death is an individual experience
We cannot die on behalf of someone else or take their place—I would be asking for volunteers if that were the case. We all have to meet with death, face-to-face, at some time. As a young scholar in boarding school, back in the days when we were caned[1] for our indiscretions, we would queue up to be 'jacked'. It was always a dynamic process where the person at the front of the queue was taken into the privacy of the games room and—whack, whack, whack. They would leave the room highly motivated, wide-eyed, and rubbing their posteriors.

Even more impressive was the wrangling that went on in the queue, where boys near the front would surrender their position and move to the back of the line. But it would not matter where you were in the queue or how many times

---
[1] While this may seem archaic and cruel, no animals were injured in the process and we all lived to tell the tale with embellishments and laughter, and perhaps behaviour modification for a while.

you changed position, you were still going to meet with your own personalised, individual version of the 'whack'.

In the same way, it does not matter where we are in the queue of life and how many times we might change position, our meeting with death is a personalised and private affair destined to happen. We may fear the 'whack' of death due to the reaction of others, but my experience has been that each person individually finds a way to cope.

Death touches many lives

The implications of our death will affect many, many people, starting with those we love and who love us. Our death affects society, friends, family, work colleagues and, eventually, the butcher, baker and candlestick maker who no longer have an opportunity to do business with us. At the extreme is the government, who will no longer be able to tax you when you are dead. You will be sorely missed...

Death can be kind

For some people, there comes a time when life is no longer a gift, when the body is broken and wracked with pain and suffering, and death is a welcomed friend.

Death only happens on one day in your life

Of all the days you get to live, death only happens on one of them. The rest of our time belongs to us. Being fixated on avoiding death when we should be getting on with life is a common mistake people make. It is better to be prepared for death, so that you can get on with life without distraction.

Death is a spiritual event
Each life ends with us going to meet with our God. It is a personal one-on-one meeting. At the point of death, our spirit leaves our lifeless body for *that* moment of truth where we all find out about our belief systems.

Death has a low standard—you cannot fail
Death has no great expectations. Everyone passes the test and there are no failures. The good, the bad, the ugly, the brave, the timid—all make the grade. When we die, we join the majority, all those who have gone before us. Everyone has passed with flying colours. The good news about dying is that you will be just fine when the time comes.

The thing about death is that the time often comes too quickly. If only we had another year or two! While we may accept that we have to die, it's hardly ever a good time. Would it help if you knew in advance the day of your death, that 12 June 2035 would be your last day? Would knowing make a difference to how you lived your life? Some might relish the thought of 'going nuts' until the day arrives, while others simply would not want to know.

Death sometimes arrives unannounced. These are difficult deaths, ones that start off as a normal day at the office and end up as a day in the morgue. They are traumatic for those left behind. Fortunately, these are more the exception than the rule, and most of us get given at least some notice of death's intention to pay us a visit. I think this is a kindness, that it is death being polite and saying, "Hey, I am heading your way soon." It gives us time to tidy up our lives and have our bags packed ready to go at the right time.

Chapter 4

The Iceberg Moment

It is easy to talk about death when it is abstract and distant. We can all cope with death quite easily on those terms, but it is a different story when it looks in our direction and we know it is on its way. This moment of reality is the 'iceberg moment'.

On 10 April 1912, the passenger liner RMS *Titanic* set sail from Southampton on its maiden voyage. It was labelled the 'unsinkable ship', and there was great celebration and excitement on the voyage to New York. Everything was just wonderful, and this was going to be the first of many memorable experiences. There was dining and laughter and an unshakeable expectation of arriving in New York.

At 11:30 pm on 14 April, all that was about to change. As the *Titanic* roared through the icy Atlantic Ocean, it bore down on an iceberg. The danger was duly reported, and immediate evasive action taken. After what seemed a glancing blow, the ship sailed on. Less than three hours later, at 2:20 am, the majestic *Titanic* slid into the icy depths of the Atlantic Ocean, claiming 1500 lives.

In the dark, unfolding chaos, the unfortunate people on the *Titanic* were forced to face the reality of their new situation and come to terms with their fate. In those three dark hours they had to transition from the joy and merriment of a maiden voyage to the possibility—and for 1500 people the reality—of death. What a disaster!

Between the iceberg moment and the sinking, those on board had limited time to figure things out. "What must we do?" "How can we escape?" These questions must have been in their minds. They needed an immediate disaster management plan, and in these circumstances, denial is often our first line of defence. Denial is an immediate ally, and we can blame no-one for first seeking consolation at the door of denial. But denial beguiles all, it makes loud promises which it cannot fulfill. It is a parachute that won't open, a life raft with a hole, a lifebuoy without a rope.

Denial comes in many shapes and forms. For those on the *Titanic*, their first denial was absolute. This form of denial refuses to see, listen or act. It shouts that nothing has happened. The ship did not hit the iceberg. There is no damage. We can continue as before. The ship is unsinkable!

This denial is so audacious that even in the face of overwhelming evidence—such as the literal sinking of the ship—it will hold true to its story. It is an irrational and delusional fiend. It insists that the party must go on and to do anything else should be punished.

This denial is blind and threatens to destroy all who challenge it. It never concedes, but because it is so profoundly deluded, it is quickly dismissed by most rational people. This is the denial that allows people to grow unimaginably big, smelly and festering cancers and remain blissfully unaware of the problem.

This makes room for the second denial. This denial sees and accepts the new reality, but refuses to accept any responsibility or need to act. It plays down the new reality as being irrelevant and nothing to worry about.

This denial says things such as:

- Yes, there is a hole in the boat, but it is a small hole, and it can be fixed.
- The hole is in one of the forward compartments, but they are secure so all will be well.
- This ship is built to be unsinkable so no need to worry.
- They will get someone to fix it, I am sure this happens a lot.
- They will get lifeboats, or a ship will save us. Relax, don't worry.

When it comes to dying, this denial is the most commonly used coping strategy. There is acceptance that we will die and there is no need to worry about this:

- It will happen later.
- It happens to other people.
- They will find a cure.

- Everything will be ok.
- No need to change a thing—keep calm and carry on.
- She'll be right, mate.

It is a cheerful fellow, this denial, but so very irresponsible. Like the first one, this denial prevents any transition.

The third denial is the one that sees and acts, but the action is misdirected, and because of this the real issue is avoided. It can be a master showman, a prestidigitator of note. It will get everyone to sing the national anthem while the ship is sinking or set everyone to rearranging the chairs on the deck, rather than directing their efforts to solving the real problem.

It is this denial that will accept a terminal diagnosis, only to keep trying to fight it to the bitter end. All that energy and effort is directed at solving the wrong problem. It is this misdirection and 'call to arms' that prevents people from focussing on the real issue—finding a way to come to terms with death.

This third denial can be a noble cause. Typically, it is where we see the pursuit of alternative therapies, magic cures, faith healing or a curative diet. By this time, the standard medical options have failed. "But what do they know after all?" Don't mess with this denial if it is on a crusade, it can be just as nasty as its first cousin.

While these three denials may seem innocent enough, and can all easily look like our best friend, they never are.

Denial is a thief. It robs the dying of the precious time and energy that are needed to prepare for death. It also robs people of knowing and accepting the truth. It comes at a great cost.

I remember Trudy, a patient who was diagnosed with Stage 4 colorectal cancer. Everything seemed to be fine after bowel surgery for her colon cancer until, after many years, she developed a spot on her lung. The cancer had come back, and because it was an isolated spot and had reappeared after so many years, she underwent a surgical resection. Everything was looking good, until the discovery that the cancer had spread to her liver and ultimately, her brain. Despite an unfavourable prognosis, Trudy refused to accept that she was dying.

Her denial could not stop her dying, but it did:

- alienate her husband and children, ultimately breaking down family relationships because the family needed to prepare for her death, and she denied them this
- shut down communication; she would not speak to anyone who did not buy into her denial
- affect her choices in life, because she went on a crusade and spent her time in death-defying activity rather than life affirming choices
- prevent her preparing for death—there is a lot to get done

- fail to live up to its promises. Trudy died alone, rather than in the company of those who loved her.

Denial can sometimes masquerade as kindness. Mandy's father had been diagnosed with terminal brain cancer, and she explained how they "protected him" from his diagnosis by refusing to talk about it. Whenever he brought it up in conversation, they would intentionally shut him down with kind words, such as "it will be ok" and "you will be fine; you're not going to die." This seemingly kind approach to helping, actually hindered him. He was denied the opportunity to prepare for death and the chance to say goodbye on his terms.

I know that denial is often only a phase, and it can be a good initial coping mechanism. In my career, I have found that persistent denial is a destructive force that stops people from preparing for a good death. I say this in the sense that death doesn't only affect the person dying, but also everyone on the journey. Denial shuts the door to acceptance, and in dying, that door needs to be open. There should be open conversations, moments of laughter amid the tears, reflection, celebration, sharing, and above all, an opportunity to love and be loved. For all these reasons denial must be defeated and sometimes this takes time.

There will be an iceberg moment for all of us, whether in our life or in the life of someone we love. This may potentially be the worst day in our life. It will come with a terrible shock. It will be a mind-numbing blow and there is no way to soften it so that it does not hurt. At that moment, death is no longer abstract and theoretical, it has become a reality, and everything changes. Our comfortable and safe lives are disrupted irreversibly. We are forced into a new painful reality, and we need to find a way to cope.

It takes time to digest this new reality after that iceberg moment.

- It can't be true.
- It is not possible.
- There has to be some mistake, I am too young to die.
- This is not God's plan.

Denial can give you something to hold onto at first, but then what? If your ship is sinking, you need a plan that addresses the real problem.

Chapter 5

The Changing Narrative

When we become aware of death's approach, we are obliged to undertake a painful journey of transition. This transition starts at the point of being in good health, where illness and death are *impossible* considerations. You cannot die from illness if you are in perfect health.

On the other side of this transition is the certainty of death, where health and wellness are *impossible* considerations. It is difficult to avoid death when death is not avoiding you. Moving from an expectation of living to an expectation of dying is a big ask and a long journey. It is the most difficult thing you'll ever need to do because it involves so many things along the way. This is why death education is so important. We cannot get from one point to the other without help or a roadmap of some kind.

Some people refuse to acknowledge this transition. They remain in a state of denial, and even when life is out of sight, they refuse to consider the nearness of death. It is understandable, and they cannot be judged for holding on to everything in this life, but it is not sustainable. At some point, with or without our consent, death will visit. Even with the best intentions of ignoring death, most people are forced along this pathway of transition by their changing physical condition.

For some people, the transition from perfect health to death happens instantly. They leave home in good health and in good spirits and do not return at night because of a catastrophic event, such as a motor vehicle accident or a massive heart attack. There is no transition period or time to get ready for death. There are no goodbyes, affirmations of love or opportunities for reconciliation. Death may be instantaneous, and from one perspective, this may seem to be a good way to go—dead, and you don't even know it. The good thing about this sudden transition is that it requires no effort; it is over before it begins. But any death affects more than the person who has died; it affects a whole family or community. In my experience, these instant deaths are the most chaotic, and they leave the deepest and longest scars of bereavement and loss in those who are left behind.

The process of transition is called dying. It is a verb, an action word. Dying is a dynamic and ever-changing process, and there are important things to know about how it works. There are challenging physical changes associated with dying. Knowing them means that they can be managed at the right time and in the right way. There are also strong emotions involved in dying, and it is important to find shelter from this storm.

The Changing Narrative

Dying is a spiritual event, and we cannot provide death education without touching on matters of eternity. There are also many practical things to know about and to do in the process of dying. It takes a lot of effort; dying is exhausting.

Dying is worse than being dead. Being dead is, in many ways, the easy part because it's all over then. There are no more responsibilities once you are dead, and the suffering has come to an end. Nothing more can be done or undone past the point of death. The final whistle has blown, the game is over, and the scoreboard is unchangeable.

Because dying is hard work, it may seem easier to quit while you are ahead, but there is no way to quit. There is no way to escape; we all have to go through it.

The way to get through all the aspects of dying is the same way we get through other big tasks in life—by taking one small step at a time. We won't get there if we do not take that *first step*, and it is this first step of transition that is often the most difficult one. We can only take that step if we feel safe. And it will depend on our narrative and how we allow it to change.

As doctors, the one thing we hate doing the most is giving patients bad news. And the worst news to give is that there is an incurable or terminal illness. In my work as an oncologist, I often have to tell patients that their cancer has returned and that they have an incurable disease. The narrative that we all hope for—that all is well, and we have cured the cancer—is no longer valid. The narrative changes when we have an iceberg moment. What do you say when this happens?

How do you tell the captain of the *Titanic* that he has hit an iceberg? Do you meekly say, "Excuse me Captain, I think there is a tiny problem"? Or do you say, "Oh crap! We have just struck an enormous iceberg"? Whatever you say won't change the fact that the ship is sinking, but it will change the way you cope with the ship sinking. The way we convey bad news sets us up for how we manage the disaster.

We could say nothing. We could get someone else to say something—that is usually the easiest. But most people have the same strategy, and it ends up that no one says anything.

There can be no good news when there is bad news, and when there is bad news, we need a way to say it with honesty and compassion. Platitudes like "she'll be right, mate" or "everything is going to be okay" do not work if they are not true. When there is change in the narrative, we need to let all those involved know, so that they have time to adjust and prepare.

I recently had to tell my good friend Bill that he had stage four incurable cancer. I had been involved in his care and, as a friend, I kept a close eye on his progress and results while he was receiving care at a large academic hospital. I remember looking at his Positron Emission Tomography (PET) scan images and feeling the dull shock as I tried to digest the evidence of the new large incurable cancer in his lungs. In that moment of truth, you can only say, "Oh no! Please, no!"

When I looked at the scan, I knew that this year would be his last birthday, that his future grandchildren would never know their 'Pops', and that he would never get to see his son graduate as a lawyer. I knew that his wife was going to be left alone, and that she might not manage too well on her own. I knew the disease trajectory and the associated symptoms of the illness. As a doctor, how can you not also shed tears for what is being taken away?

How do you tell your friend that the narrative has changed?
When do you communicate that the narrative has changed?

These are the hardest conversations you'll ever need to have. As doctors we should know that we need to break the news gently and slowly over time. We need to be honest, but sometimes poetic licence is required, so you start the conversation at the *right time* and continue the conversation at another time. We need to listen and allow space for the conversation to flow in the direction it needs to. We know that we are not required to fix the problem; we are required to be there, to be with the person who has to suffer terrible news.

We know that breaking bad news is best done in sessions, so it is good to fire a warning shot: "There is a problem." This allows the brain to start working on the problem.

Bill:

> *There are some things that worry me on your recent PET scan. Do you mind coming to see me so that we can discuss the results?*

Bill came to see me, and the conversation continued. What I knew, he didn't want to know. It is always important to get the narrative right and to provide honest reality, but in a way that is digestible. It has to be kind, compassionate and provide hope. But it also has to be truthful.

And for Bill, it would create the same problem. How do you tell your spouse that you have terminal cancer? What do you say to your children when you know that your prognosis is limited to months? How do you break the news to your parents that their child is going to die before them?

The husband to his wife:

> *I saw the doctor today, and he was concerned about some of my tests. I'll check back with him.*

To the adult child:

> *I have been feeling a bit unwell, and I am going to see the doctor on Thursday.*

These initial conversations buy time, and they pave the way for the next conversation. They allow us to formulate a plan and a strategy for what we are going to say. And what we say sets the tone for the rest of the story. Without giving it some thought, it can all go terribly wrong. Perhaps the worst comment I have heard came from one of the participants in a research group. During the narrative about their prognosis and diagnosis, they were told, "Don't buy any green bananas", implying there would not be time to see them ripen. How awful!

It takes courage to talk about a changed narrative, but talking about it is, in many ways, an opportunity to care and express love for the person who has to carry the burden of the changed narrative. It takes courage to tell and be told about the road that leads to the end of your life.

The way we look down that road will depend on the next narrative.

***

In the next narrative, the old story has ended and a new story is needed. Its narrative will determine the rest of this journey. If it tells the story that death is unbearable suffering, then it will be unbearable. Each step away from life and closer to death will be harder than the last. It will be an uphill battle with impossible last days because that is what the narrative says death is like. However, if the narrative tells us that death is no more than going to sleep or the doorway to the next great adventure in heaven, then we will find that each step along the way is possible. It is important to pick your narrative carefully.

It is not uncommon in eulogies to hear the words, "He lost the battle with cancer." This seems a brave narrative, and it conjures up images of heroic victory. The reality, however, is that with cancer or any other terminal illness, comes certain defeat. The narrative of fighting a losing battle is a difficult one. There is never downtime, and the whole journey to the end of life can be exhausting. Fighting to the bitter end can be very bitter indeed. If you view the journey for the rest of your life as a war, it will require ongoing resources of aggression and anger. There are no truces, and there is no place for fun. Fun means failure. As much as this is a bold narrative, it is not a kind one.

Your narrative will be your most important road map going forward. It is made up of the permissions and directions you give yourself for how you are going to live the rest of your life. You don't have to wait for an iceberg moment to choose this narrative. You don't have to base your narrative on the experiences of others. Your story is not set in concrete; you are allowed to change your mind about what you want it to be. And it is *your* story—you own it, so why not make it a good one?

Perhaps the best way to think about it is to consider your life as a book filled with chapters. There was the birth chapter, then your early childhood chapter. There were stormy adolescent chapters, the marriage chapter, the 'children' chapters, work achievements and promotion chapters. The retirement and ageing chapters and illness chapters may lie ahead, but there could still be many adventures before you get to the final chapter and the end of the story.

How do you want your story to end? We often assume that the end is going to be all bad, but there is the choice to make it as good as we possibly can. It must be based on reality and honesty, but it can also include the expectation of outrageous fun. If you are going to have a hip replacement, then go for the bionic enhanced hip option that gives you an unfair advantage and lets you win at tennis. If you are going to need a wheelchair, get the one with racing wheels. If you are going to end up bedridden, make sure your bed is in a 5-star resort, next to a tropical pool. If you need a funeral, make sure it has a pink theme with marshmallows for everyone. Why do boring? Make your story as fun as it can be.

I caught up with my friend Bill and told him about the scan results and told him the truth of his condition in the gentlest way possible. My friend struggled with the news, but he had a good narrative. He was realistic about his diagnosis and prognosis. He tried immunotherapy with the expectation that it was going to work. It worked for six months, and then he died peacefully surrounded by his family, and protected by his narrative that was based on faith with an expectation of heaven.

My role as his friend was not to prevent him from dying, but to help him on this bumpy road. I was there to keep him company, to pick him up when he fell, and to help him complete his journey. We were not going off to war to fight battles. We were doing the final lap in life and enjoying the journey.

If you need to start preparing for the transition from life to death, why not make the journey as easy as you can by creating a narrative of hope? We are not always in control of our narrative, and sometimes, with the best of intentions, our narrative has to change. That's okay, we can always start a new story if the one we have no longer serves its purpose. The only prerequisite for your narrative is that it must be based on the current reality. And for that we need to look at the reality of death and dying.

We have to start with the question of why we die and the problem of getting old.

Chapter 6

The Death Code, Ageing & Why We Die

Beware! You have been programmed. While this may seem like the plot of an elaborate science fiction movie, it is part of everyday life. We have all been programmed by our DNA (deoxyribonucleic acid) genetic code. This code determines whether you look like your father or your mother. Your DNA comes pre-loaded with the specifications for your eye colour, your height, your temperament, your abilities and your probable lifespan. Packed away in the code are all the good and the not-so-good things about you.

In medicine, we ask for a family history, not because we are curious about what your parents have been up to, but so we can know the weak points of your genetic makeup. Did your parent have heart disease? Well, chances are you will have heart disease, too. If they are diabetics, you better watch your sugar intake. However, the family history can only offer hints of what may be ahead. You are not totally dependent on your parents' genes. You can relax; you won't turn into your parents. You don't fully rely on their code; you get to bring along your own. Your DNA is a brand-new blend of unique genetic material. There is no one like you—you are a masterpiece.

The DNA code is wrapped up in every cell and it directs the function of each one. It is, if you like, the cell's brain. The DNA's code delivers a message that results in a specific cellular function and action. Good DNA means good messages and good function, and there are hundreds and thousands of good messages occurring every day.

It may help to picture our genetic code as the thousands and thousands of stitches in our newly knitted jumper. When we first get it, it is fresh, crisp and clean. It's immediately our favourite jumper, and we wear it day and night. Over the years, the jumper becomes frayed and worn. Like everything else in life, it gets older and wears out. There are holes where 'life happened'. The jumper may have been snagged on a nail or subject to excessive stretching and pulling, so it is no longer perfect, but it does the job. It remains our favourite piece of clothing. The holes eventually get bigger, the stiches unravel more, and there comes a time when we must, with great reluctance, get rid of the tatty old jumper. The same principle of decay occurs in all aspects of life: cars rust, wood rots, clothes become threadbare, and even the immovable landscape changes over time.

In a similar way, and for the same reasons, our pristine DNA degenerates over time. What starts off crisp and fresh and new at birth soon becomes worn and tired. While DNA has an amazing ability to repair itself, this also eventually shows wear and tear. Soon, like the jumper, the DNA has a few snags and rips and holes. These are made worse by a range of factors, including alcohol, poor diet, cigarette smoke, radiation and poor lifestyle choices. These normal everyday assaults on our DNA eventually cause enough DNA damage to affect our function. First, the DNA is damaged, then the code gets damaged, the messages get corrupted, and finally cellular function is affected. This malfunction of the cell causes the chronic degenerative illnesses associated with ageing.

For some, our genes increase our likelihood of cancer, for others it may be a stroke or a heart attack or, for others, simply old age. This is not being negative. It is being realistic about your chances based on your DNA. Our DNA has a powerful say in things, but it is not the only factor in life. We can protect our DNA to some extent by making good lifestyle choices, but there is no protection against misfortune or stupidity. Drink driving, for example, is an unnecessary cause of early death. This can be caused by stupidity if we drive while inebriated, or by misfortune if we are hit by a drunk driver.

At the end of life, assuming we survive all the other risks, we must contend with old age. This is mostly due to our deteriorating genetic code. There are many theories about why we age, and the most attractive is that we run out of DNA. Every time a cell replicates itself it loses a small fragment of DNA found at the tip of the DNA strand. This important fragment gets smaller and smaller until there is nothing of it left, and then the DNA fails. This happens after about 50 cell divisions, and it explains why cells die. Cells don't last forever so they need to be replaced, but they can only be replaced so many times.

In his compelling book, *Lifespan,* Dr David A. Sinclair discusses aging and why we age. He believes it is not only our DNA, but the supporting genetic structures (called epigenes) that matter. These structures regulate our genes and with time our cells lose their identity because of epigenetic loss. Brain cells forget that they are brain cells, lung cells forget they are lung cells. Our cellular function gets watered down rather than ending abruptly. In his book, Dr Sinclair argues for living not only longer, but better. This is exciting research suggesting that the effects of ageing can be somewhat reversed. But what then?

If we could magically reset our age by 10 years, and do this over and over again until the age of 1000, would it make us happy? Even if we could solve the secrets of biological function and live another 100 years, we would still end up with the problem of our mortality. We all come back to the same place eventually: growing old.

It is difficult to grow old. It is a journey of diminishing returns and greater losses. There is the loss of sight and hearing. Smell is diminished. Muscle strength decreases and mobility becomes an issue. Falls are more common, and eventually, the dreaded wheelie walker becomes a part of the everyday shuffle. Mental processes slow down for many. Everything takes longer, and by the age of 80, it is a miracle for some to still be driving. Sex is a distant memory. Chewing requires a spare set of teeth. Getting dressed and undressed requires meticulous strategic planning. With age comes the loss of independence and a need to rely on the care of others. The great unmentioned loss in ageing is of loved ones and friends who die and leave an ever-increasing void of loneliness.

If you think it is easy to be old, spend some time speaking to an older person. Ask your local 95-year-old how things are going. Visit the nearest aged care facility and have dinner with the residents and get a feel of what it's like to be old. If you are still super enthusiastic about living to 100, let me know why.

This pessimism about getting very, very old is obviously not true for everybody. There are amazing centenarians who keep on keeping on. They have unbelievable genetics and epigenetics, and they are often inspirational in the way they live. There are very few who make it past 105 years, and there are almost none who have made it past 110 years old. Even for the best of us there comes a time to call it quits. There comes a time when it is an advantage to die.

This sounds blunt, but it should not be seen in a negative way. At the end of a good life, we should all be ready for a good death. If you could live for as long as you like, what would you choose? Perhaps it is an unfair question because we all want to live forever.

It may be better to ask instead, "If your father or spouse could live as long as *you* like, what would you choose?" This puts the need for dying in a different perspective. We know that there's a 'best before date' for all of us and, once we pass this date, life becomes sour just like the milk in the fridge.

We do not want the ones we love to die—we love them too much. Equally, we do not want them to live forever because we love them too much. We have a bitter choice to make because longevity comes with an increasing cost. Most people say they want quality over quantity of life, but we all really want both. This option is not on the menu.

Our genetic code may have given us our advantage or disadvantage in life. Not everyone can be an Olympian, not everyone can be an opera singer. Not everyone can live to 100 years old. We make the best of what we have. Although the length of our life may be uncertain, we hope the ride will be a good one. And when the ride is over, may we be ready to accept the truth that we meet with death.

If this thought still gives you the heebie-jeebies, think of it as no more than a passing inconvenience for now. There is still a lot of ground to cover, and the next step on the journey is to understand what goes on when the body finally malfunctions.

Chapter 7

Physical Death

It is difficult to define physical death. From day one, death has been lethal. It leaves no one untouched: it is estimated that for each person alive now, between 15 and 30 people have already died. Based on these numbers, it means that up to 200 billion people have already died. We are not the only people to die, nor the first people to die. When we die, we join the majority of people—those who have already died.

There is never a quiet day for death, death is always busy. But what exactly is death?

Most people understand it as the permanent end of the vital functions of a person or organism.

Another definition found online: "The state of being dead." Well, top marks for that comment.

In Australia, the legal definition of death, if we use Section 41 of the *Human Tissue Act 1982* (Vic) as our guide, states a person has died when there has been an irreversible cessation of circulation of blood in the body of a person or irreversible cessation of all function of the brain of the person.

These definitions do not really help us understand death; we should first consider life, and then define death as the absence of life.

It is easy to define 'life', because it is characterised by a response to a stimulus. If you poke or prod something that is alive, it will respond. We might have tested this as children by poking a biological specimen we thought was dead, only to be startled when it responded to our touch. I can think of many flapping fish or wriggling worms that seemed quite safe and dead, until they were touched.

We learn about this response to stimulus as step one of first aid and CPR. If someone looks dead and unresponsive, go up to them and try to get a response. If they respond to a loud noise or a well-placed pinch, they are alive and, depending on the circumstances and the magnitude of your stimulus, *you* may be lucky to be alive. If you've ever tested this theory by using water on a sleeping sibling, you'll know what I mean by 'lucky to be alive'.

Life is vibrant and it always responds to stimuli, which are not always as obvious as a bucket of water or a well-placed pinch. In the human body there are many stimuli that automatically and secretly happen deep in the brain to keep us alive. Subconsciously, our brains remind our hearts to beat and our lungs to breathe. These stimuli do not require our conscious direction or permission to happen. We can sleep safely without having to think about breathing. Our hearts beat without us needing a metronome. Even if we were unconscious and unable to respond to a prod or poke, our respiratory and cardiac reflexes would faithfully continue working. They are the last ones we lose when life is ending.

There is also one other handy non-vital reflex that is worth mentioning: our pupillary light reflex. It requires no conscious thought. If you shine a bright light into someone's eye, their pupil will automatically constrict and become smaller. It is fun to do this experiment, provided the participant is willing and the light is not blinding. This reflex is also lost when life ends. When a pupil does not respond to light, the person is either dead or blind. Which of the two they are is usually obvious because those who are blind will loudly protest if they are being prepared for burial.

Death can be thought of as the irreversible end of response to all stimuli. The pupil of a dead person will remain fixed and dilated, no matter how much light you shine in the eye. The dead heart will not respond to stimulus, no matter how much CPR you give. The lungs will not restart the respiratory reflex, no matter how much ventilation you provide. Exactly where this becomes irreversible is a point of contention in resuscitation. There is a time when you have to stop and declare that death has occurred. The irreversible has happened.

What exactly happens at the point of death? When is life permanently extinguished? As a young medical student, I was asked to look after Jacob, a homeless man who was dying and had been brought into the emergency department. As a junior there was not much I could do, but I was asked to take care of him. I think my supervisor saw it as an easy way to put me out of the way in a safe space where I could do little harm. I was able to spend time with Jacob as he died and, while I had little to offer this man, being able to sit with him was a gift to me.

Jacob was provided with pain control and hooked up to an electrocardiogram (ECG) monitor (an ECG measures heart activity) and an automatic blood pressure device. These scientifically recorded his vital functions. At first, he had some response to stimuli and made some groans and noises when I spoke to him. As he died, he became less conscious. Mild stimuli caused him to respond but with movement that lacked purpose. His speech was no longer discernible, only unintelligible groans. These responses diminished quickly.

Over the space of a few hours, Jacob became unresponsive. He no longer responded to external stimuli. I could shake him or pinch him and he would not move or react in anyway. His breathing changed and became irregular. His blood pressure dropped, and his ECG tracing slowed down to 60 beats/minute. His erratic breathing finally stopped and his heart slowed down to 40 beats/minute, then 20, until finally he 'flat-lined' showing no electrical activity from his heart.

His pupils were dilated and remained fixed. He was clinically dead, and I had been able to witness this transition from life to death. While this is not a remarkable story in that it is commonplace for people to die, it did allow me time to think about the process and time of death. It is not always as straightforward as it was with Jacob.

Some questions remain about exactly when and how we die. There are some grey areas, because there are some circumstances where you may be essentially dead, but not quite irreversibly so. Who knows exactly where that line is? Are you dead if you are frozen with no pulse or respiration and show no response to any stimuli? Not necessarily. You have to be warm to be dead. People who have been clinically dead and frozen have been successfully thawed and resuscitated and have lived to tell the tale.

Are you dead if your body functions are preserved, but your brain shows no signs of activity, or brain death has occurred? This can be a very difficult question when someone is in the grey area between mostly and completely dead, and no one can make up their mind. This was the terrible tragedy of the Terri Schiavo saga. Her story made it to *Time* magazine and involved a right-to-die legal case in the United States from 1998 to 2005.

The story started with Terri's cardiac arrest, where she required resuscitation and was left with permanent brain damage, resulting in what is known as a persistent vegetative state. She was clearly not dead; she was breathing and her heart was beating, but there was no other response to stimulus. Her husband wanted her to be declared dead so that they could remove the feeding tube required to keep her alive. Her parents wanted her to be given the care she required to stay alive, hoping against hope in this terrible situation. After a fierce legal contest, which would eventually even involve the then US President George W. Bush, it was determined that her feeding tube was to be removed on 18 March 2005. Terri died on 31 March 2005.

Another remarkable story involved Jayne Soliman, who 'died' of a brain haemorrhage while she was pregnant. Despite being declared brain dead, she was kept alive long enough to have a Caesarean section and safely deliver her child. This medical miracle once again blurs the lines between life and death.

Death is so evident after the event. The clinical signs used to confirm death are the absence of breathing, heartbeat, brain activity and light reflex. It was easy to see that Jacob had died after his death, but while he was dying there was no way of definitively establishing whether he was still partly alive or mostly dead.

After death, some physiological processes still run in the background. Organs like the heart, lungs and kidneys are still viable for organ transplantation. The final physical changes before all function ceases are like a car that continues to skid along the highway after the brakes have been applied. It is easy to know when the car has finally come to a dead stop. It is far more uncertain when the driver applied the brakes.

Reflecting on Jacob, I wanted to know the instant of his death. Put another way, when was it that his life left him? This begs the next question: what exactly makes us alive? If it is only a matter of biology, we should ultimately be able to conquer death and live forever by providing optimal biological support and the replacement of malfunctioning cells.

There is a mystery about death that is explained by spiritual existence. There is evidence that, at the time of death, our spirit leaves our physical body. This spiritual event is like being unplugged from the power grid and results in our immediate death. Some processes may continue to run for a while, but they are token physiological processes, which wind down and stop soon after our spiritual-physical interaction ends. We will discuss this amazing possibility in near death experiences.

For now, it is enough to say that up to the time of death there is a lot going on. After death there is nothing—it is quiet, and it is peaceful. There are the expected feelings of loss and bereavement that follow when a life ends, and those left behind still have tasks ahead of them, but the one who has died is now at rest. May this be in peace.

Chapter 8

Physical Aspects of Dying

We cannot get to death unless we die, and this takes some effort. It is not something we can practise or perfect, we all get just one go at it, and all we can hope for is a smooth landing.

When I lived in New Zealand, a friend who was an instructor pilot invited me to come along on some 'joy rides' in Dannevirke. I was very excited about flying. We had spoken about all the theory of flying and windspeed and bearing, and as a couch-potato pilot, I felt ready to experience the real thing.

Dannevirke Airport is not bustling. It is a strip of dirt with a little building. There was the plane, instructor and student. Being naïve, I invited my son along for the flight and the two of us squeezed into the back of the plane. The pilot and instructor duly filed into the front seats and away we went, zooming along the airstrip to become airborne and free.

It was at about this time that I realised that the pilot

was, in fact, nothing of the sort. He was actually a scholar training to be a pilot, and he was practising the most basic of skill sets: take-off and landing. In reality, he did not know much about flying. The instructor *did* know a lot about flying, but he wasn't flying the plane so there was much to learn on the way down.

When you land, there are apparently a few things to consider, such as airspeed, angle of approach and cross winds, and there are several things to keep checking, such as flaps and wheels. There is also gravity threatening to pull you into the ground at an uncalculated and alarming speed, in what is commonly known as a crash.

The novice pilot manoeuvred the plane, bringing it into line despite the wind swaying the tail to and fro, and thankfully, we came in to land quite safely. I'd never been more pleased to be on the ground, but this feeling was short-lived. The novice gunned the engine, and we took off again. Circuits! We were doing circuits. I soon had to endure the same anxiety and distress all over again. I made my intentions of abandoning the plane clearly known, and I vowed never again. Once was enough.

When it comes down to it, flying and dying share many similarities. Doctors are the instructors. They know a lot, but they are not holding the controls. The person who is dying is the one in charge of the process, but they are only a novice and don't really know what they are doing. Their loved ones are the passengers in the back hoping for the nail-biting best. All the while, there are instruments showing the crosswinds, angles of approach, wind speed, flaps and other things that constantly need checking as the runway approaches. Thankfully, when it comes to dying, we only do it once.

There are many things that influence how we die, and for each of us the journey will be different. It can depend on our reserves and general fitness. If you are older, have a long list of medical conditions or don't have access to good medical care, chances are that dying will be over sooner. It can also depend on the diagnosis. Some cancers have shorter descents than others, whereas motor neuron disease and chronic illnesses have long flight plans, and the landing seems to go on forever.

Pain is a common threat, and pain management is an essential skill. For cancer, the other crosswinds are weight loss, fatigue, occasional breathlessness, nausea and, if relevant, the side effects of treatment. Each new symptom requires an adjustment to the fine-tuning of the final approach before landing. Each disease has its own unique challenge and, when the time comes, the best advice is to ask your doctor what to expect and how to manage the symptoms to ensure there is a safe landing.

Regardless of the diagnosis, the flights will all end in much the same way. The plane is kept level, the speed is reduced, and with practice, there is the lightest of touchdowns—hardly anything at all. In the final approach, there are several common symptoms (particularly from a cancer perspective) that should be expected. Knowing about these makes the landing more predictable and perhaps a little less frightening. Regardless of the nature and course of disease, the symptoms at the end of life are similar. This is a fragile and precious time, when one should complete the final checks and commit to the final touchdown.

Common symptoms

The following are common symptoms at the end of life.

Increasing fatigue and weariness

Illness uses up energy, and everyday activities become difficult as this energy is depleted. Even getting up out of bed is exhausting and often no longer possible. Assistance is required with all activities, including getting to and from the bathroom. Sleep is a good friend. Visitors can be a burden, and at this stage, there is no longer the vitality to do the things that may have been left undone. There is simply no more fuel left in the tank.

Lack of interest in surroundings

The attractiveness of life is lost, and hobbies or activities once enjoyed are no longer appealing. Watching football on television or reading a favourite novel is not worth the effort. Assets worth millions of dollars are no longer important. Everyday things that used to be of value no longer hold any value. The runway lies ahead, and the focus is no longer on the scenery but on the landing.

Loss of appetite

Eating is no longer important. Food loses its flavour and appeal. Often background nausea contributes to the poor appetite. Eating is mostly a feeble attempt to appease the needs of the family who insist on it, but the body no longer needs food. This is often the biggest battleground as family members try to prevent death from approaching—they know that if you don't eat you will die, and they hope that if you do eat, death won't be rude and interrupt your meal.

Increased confusion and restlessness

It feels as if the body no longer fits properly—like wearing a pair of ill-fitting shoes or a scratchy woollen garment. The result is restlessness and fidgeting as the discomfort of illness increases. In addition, subject to the chemical changes associated with dying, the brain becomes increasingly confused. Increased drowsiness, confusion and impaired consciousness are common as death approaches.

Fasten your seatbelts—the dying phase

When the body is dying, there is a whole lot going on. But for the dying brain, there is less and less happening as consciousness is diminished. Those dying are mostly unaware of the drama that is unfolding. Pain can be managed, and the dying person should not be suffering. Syringe drivers are introduced to provide effective pain control and *not*, as incorrectly believed by some, to hasten death. Death is already at the door, and it needs no invitation.

Spectators are often distressed by the changes to the body in the last 48-hour period. Emotions run high. There is great uncertainty about what to expect and when to expect it. The time for goodbyes has passed. Often people think that they will have time to have a final chat and conversation. Usually by now it is too late. But, as always, there are exceptions.

Sometimes, people who are on their death bed miraculously revive, sit up and are the life of the party for a brief period—only to relapse and die in the next few days. This is inexplicable, but it has been reported enough times for us to know that there sometimes is a brief honeymoon phase before dying. This is known as terminal lucidity, and if it were not such a solemn time, it could be quite amusing. It may last for a few hours, as in the following example.

> Poor old aunt Edna was unconscious and ready to die. She was surrounded by her family, who were expecting the worst at any moment. The doctors had given her hours to live when—BANG, she opened her eyes and asked for a pickled sandwich and when her son, Allan, would be arriving.
>
> What started out to be a death vigil, quickly escalated into a party. Edna never looked better—mainly because she could not have possibly looked worse. She chatted and carried on. It was the miracle all had been praying for! The doctors were embarrassed by missing this recovery, and the family were all frustrated that they had made the 100 kilometre round trip to see poor Edna, who seemed to be in the best of health.
>
> As quickly as all this had started, Edna lapsed back into a coma and died in the next few days.

At the time of death, everything that can go wrong in the body is going wrong. The kidneys don't work, so there is no urine, or only a small dark trickle. The liver doesn't work, and the combined toxin build-up from the liver and kidneys results in increased confusion and drowsiness. Small bleeding spots are seen in the skin. The heart cannot pump properly, and the hands and feet become cold and mottled blue in colour. Blood pressure drops. The hands and feet can be puffy. These changes are cumulative and progressive. As organs fail, they result in further organ failure. A cascade of disasters affect the brain and finally the heart.

The failure of the brain deserves a special mention. It is time for touchdown.

The brain shuts down

The brain is an amazing organ. It regulates all the bodily functions. It can take a light signal and transform it into an image that makes sense so we can see. It can coordinate the movement of the throat, lips, lungs and voice box to make sounds so that we can talk and have language. It can pick up soundwaves and translate them into meaningful messages so we can hear. It enables us to make purposeful, directed movement. If, for example, you wanted to get a coffee, the brain would coordinate all the activities and planning to make that happen. We take this simple task for granted, but if you break it down into its components, making a coffee is an amazing feat.

When we go through the process of dying, the activities we take for granted are progressively lost. Initially, confusion and disorientation are common. Our sense of person: "Who am I?" Of place: "Where am I?" And of time: "What time is it now and what day?" are all lost.

Next, the higher thought functions are lost. These include our language function and the ability to form words, so that all that is left to us are meaningless moans and incoherent mumblings. Planned movement is lost, and our movements become random and purposeless.

Gradually, the response to external stimuli is lost. In the coma stage, bowel and bladder control are no longer possible, and the dying person has accidents. The bed gets soiled, and this can be very distressing for the carers if they do not understand what is happening. They cannot understand why Dad has now soiled his sheets.

Soon, the brain can no longer regulate the automatic subconscious things we take for granted. Finally, the regulation of breathing and the airways is lost. Breathing patterns change and become irregular. Fast shallow breaths are followed by slow breaths, and long gaps appear between the breaths. These gaps get longer and longer until breathing stops—and then it starts again. This is known as Cheyne-Stokes Breathing. As breathing shuts down, long intervals occur between breaths with an occasional deep gasp as if the person is not getting enough air. This is not an indication that the person is suffocating, but that they are dying.

At this deep level of unconsciousness, the brain is no longer aware of the secretions in the back of the throat. They are usually automatically swallowed but this is no longer happening. Swallowing has stopped, and these secretions become obvious in breathing. They cause a wet snoring sound, and it seems that the person may be drowning in secretions. In medical terms, these sounds are known as the 'death rattle'. This is a terminal sign, and death is imminent (minutes to hours away).

The brain is dying. Consciousness is long gone. The dying person is no longer part of this world. Death is close, and at the right time, the plane lands—the flight is over, and the body is at peace. The suffering and distress of terminal illness are over. May it be a perfect landing.

The physical aspects of death are challenging. They dominate the lives of those who are dying, as well as the lives of their loved ones and carers. Physical death is easy to understand, because it is based on physiology and biology. We can measure each change in the way the body performs, do routine blood counts, categorise each symptom and manage them efficiently. From a physical perspective, we think we have this sorted.

But this is not our greatest challenge in dying. It is easy to be brave and heroic when it comes to the physical aspects of death. But heroes also cry. This pain of dying, the emotional burden of having to say goodbye and having to endure the emotional loss of death, is what makes us wince the most and dread dying more than anything else.

If we really want to be able to face death, we have to deal with our emotions.

Chapter 9

Introduction To Emotions

We do not often think about what it is exactly that bothers us the most about dying. It is easy to assume that we are most concerned about the physical aspects of dying, but this is not always true. While the physical effects of dying are not welcome, they are not necessarily our greatest concern.

We have all experienced physical suffering in some way in life. We can manage pain—we don't like it, but we can bear it. Childbirth attests to this fact. The expected physical symptoms of dying, such as pain, fatigue, shortness of breath and nausea are all manageable. These symptom-management challenges are all within the skill set of the palliative care doctors. We may be able to approach the symptoms of dying with the same enthusiasm as having a knee replacement or, for some, dental work. "It ain't going to be fun, but somehow, we will manage." The suffering during dying will pass, it does not last forever.

But there is another form of suffering we need to

contend with, and that is the feeling of loss associated with dying. This is often a far more painful experience than the physical pain associated with death. It is the emotional experience that makes dying so terrible, so unbearable, so shockingly painful for many people. It is there that we need the most help.

It is here that we also experience a transition. Unlike the physical transition that occurs in dying, this transition does not necessarily have to be a downward spiral. We do not need to be worse off emotionally because of death, and in fact some people are better off on this journey as they discover their real purpose in life.

As with all great journeys in life, our emotional journey has a starting point. This comes before the iceberg moment. By then, we already have emotional baggage and an emotional armamentarium. We must bring these with us when we cope with our loss as we look into a chasm of hopelessness where the sun never seems to shine.

This hopelessness is born of the anticipated loss of all things. In dying we not only lose our life, but also everything we have worked for. We lose all meaning, relevance and connection. For those left behind, there is the large painful hole of bereavement. For those who die, there is the threat of nothingness. In this place of hopelessness, we experience fear, guilt and the spectrum of loss and pain. It may seem as though the purpose of life is meaningless and that nothing can be saved. There are no exceptions, we are all vulnerable to these dark emotions.

Introduction to Emotions

Unlike our bodies that have no choice in taking the downward spiral of illness, our minds can stay free. In the seemingly bottomless pit of hopelessness we are presented with two choices. The first is to remain there in sorrow and hopelessness. The second is to deliberately move on from there and back towards hope. We all have this choice—to get on with dying or to get on with living.

How can this even be possible? The way out of this hopelessness is to understand the nature of emotions. They are never as real as they seem, *and we have the ability to be greater than our dark emotions.* We have access to other emotions as well, those of hope and love. To make the choice, we must be deliberate about our emotions, step back and see them for what they are. We cannot ignore them, because if we do, they will threaten to overwhelm us. We can be the masters of our emotions.

Emotions are central to our being. As humans, we live to feel. Emotions motivate us, and we are held hostage to our feelings. Our behaviour is directly linked to how things make us feel or how they potentially make us feel. We are prepared to put up with short-term pain for long-term gain.

We seek the emotion of happiness. Marketeers have known this truth for ages. We don't buy the new shoes because of the way they look, we buy them because of how they make us feel. We feel happy. We feel important. We feel sexy. We feel fulfilled in our new shoes.

The same applies to that delicious pizza at Antonio's. It is not delicious because of all the ingredients on it. The same ingredients can be found in any grocery store, but we don't really care about them. The pizza is so delicious because of how it makes us feel when we bite into that tomatoey, cheesy, mouth-watering topping, and how we feel when the flavours on this perfectly crunchy pizza base combine in our mouths. We are in emotional heaven with each bite. The ambiance of the restaurant and the delicious aroma all add to our feeling of happiness.

If we were just as hungry and had mixed all the same ingredients in exactly the same way, but ate the pizza at the courthouse, it would not taste the same even though it was the exact same pizza. We feel happier at Antonio's, and it is experiencing this happiness experience that makes us go back. Equally, if we ate the same delicious meal at Antonio's when we have just been dumped in a relationship, chances are that the pizzas there will never taste as great again.

Everything we do is emotion-based: we love, hate, feel joy and happiness, laugh, cry, and may experience fear. We buy shoes, eat pizza, drive cars, and start relationships, all because of the emotional benefits they provide. Our feelings are what make us feel alive. We can never separate ourselves from our emotions, nor would we want that.

Because emotions are so important, we need to know more about them. Here are some basic observations:

Emotions are natural and variable

Our range and depth of emotion depends on our

personalities, but we all feel them to some degree. I have a friend who, if he won a Ferrari in a car raffle, would respond with no more than a "Thank you." And, if you were to ask him how he was feeling at that moment, he would just say, "Okay." His emotions would be underwhelming, but they would be there. Then, there are others who win a $2 raffle, and you think you might need to tranquilise them to calm them down.

Emotions vary, and they can be explosive. We often see explosive emotion in sport. At the 2012 Australian Open tennis tournament, Marcos Baghdatis entertained the crowds by smashing four tennis rackets in succession—boom, boom, boom, boom! Two of them were still in their plastic wrappers, but they had no chance of surviving.

What stirs your emotions? Some people are moved to tears in response to beautiful music or sublime sunsets. Even a tough bloke can be reduced to tears on his daughter's wedding day or at the birth of a grandchild. We all feel, but not always in the same way.

Emotions are chemical

We experience emotions because of the chemistry in our brains, and there are a lot of chemical participants involved, including serotonin, dopamine, estrogen, testosterone, adrenalin and cortisol. Then there are a few of the favourite substances from outside the body, such as nicotine, alcohol, and perhaps less legal options.

Emotions are powerful

Human emotion is a powerful force. Our emotions can sometimes take us beyond our natural ability and let us do more than expected.

In sport, there are players gifted with the ability to tap into their emotions and those of the crowd and use that energy to lift their game, to get pumped up and to rise above the occasion. It is almost as if they are suddenly able to find another gear powered by emotions.

On a basic survival level, our 'fight or flight' response to adrenalin can result in superhuman feats. This happened to Lauren Kornacki when she lifted a BMW off her father who was trapped and crushed underneath. Warren 'Tiny' Everal once lifted a helicopter off a pilot injured in an accident on the set of the *Magnum PI* series. Countless inexplicable feats have been achieved while riding a surge of emotion.

Emotions are irrational

Emotions are not rational. On 29 March 2006, blind Jim Sherman entered a burning house to rescue his blind neighbour and bring her to safety. What was he thinking? People can perform acts of great bravery based on an emotional response. Clearly, saving someone's life at the risk of your own is never going to be rational.

It is the irrationality of love that allows us to ignore the faults of the ones we fall in love with. It is the same irrationality of emotion that allows hate to grow so strong in a human heart that it results in unspeakable acts, such as mass killings in US schools or suicide bombings by extremists.

Because emotions are irrational, they should be handled with care.

Emotions are affected by circumstance

What happens externally affects the chemical soup of what happens internally, and we feel emotion. How do you feel in the following circumstances:

- being late for a meeting and stuck in traffic?
- finding your lost car keys?
- holding your first grandchild?
- meeting an old friend?
- encountering an old enemy?
- losing your job?
- having a breakdown with a flat tyre?

Some of these situations may cause a powerful emotional response in us. Sometimes events in life can be so traumatic that they leave emotional scars. The unknown can also be very stressful because we have no reference points for how to behave in circumstances that are new to us, and often our default emotion is based on threat and fear. How do you feel when you are driving in a new city, and you don't know the way?

Emotions change

Our emotions can never be relied upon to stay the same, they are always capable of changing at any moment. If you watch the emotions of a toddler over any given period, you will see this ability to regularly change every few minutes. Our adult emotions can do the same, if we let them. Often, no matter how bad things might seem on one day, we wake up feeling significantly better about it in the morning. Even if nothing has actually changed about the situation, our emotions have.

It is not unusual to lie awake at night and fret under a blanket of emotion. It is worth knowing that this emotion will change, and sometimes we need to allow for that to happen. Walking away from a source of anger may allow your emotions to change enough that when you get back, you find yourself responding to the exact same thing with a completely different emotion.

Emotions make us vulnerable

Men don't cry! Or at least, that was what we were brought up to believe. Culturally, it may be wrong to express emotion because it may be seen as a sign of weakness or failure. Our emotions make us vulnerable. It is difficult to perform well if we are embarrassed or feel threatened. Do you remember asking that girl out for that first date? Or asking her father's permission to marry his daughter? It took me days of determined procrastination to pop the question to both my now-wife and her father.

Introduction to Emotions

Emotions can lie dormant

Think back to different experiences in your life. Some experiences were positive and the emotion you felt stayed with you for days. Toyota once had an advertisement campaign based on the euphoria of buying a new car with the tagline, "Are you still feeling it?"

However, some experiences are negative, and you may remember some of those. For example, the time you were punished for smoking at school, or when you got pulled over for speeding, or the day you were dumped by your boyfriend. Can you remember any of the details from the event, such as the car you were driving or the clothes you were wearing? Chances are they will be vague, but the memories and experience of the emotion you felt may still be quite real.

Suppressed emotions can erupt. They can stay with us, festering and lingering. These festering emotions are sometimes a big part of the baggage we carry with us through life. Our feelings may have been justified but they do not need to stay with us. We can get rid of them.

Emotions need to be expressed

As emotional beings, we need to express our feelings. This is easy when we attend a sporting event, such as a hockey game or a football match. With loud whooping and cheering we can let it all out. It is easy to do when there is little at stake. But expressing emotions when we are vulnerable is difficult. We are most vulnerable with those we love and want to protect and sharing our deep feelings with them is tough.

Sometimes we forget or refuse to let our emotion out, particularly when it is painful. You cannot bottle up emotion forever. Eventually, it will either leak out or explode. Punching a wall is a common cause of hand fractures in adolescent boys letting out emotion. Finding a way to express emotion safely is a skill that we can all develop. We can learn to express our emotions in therapy or through music, art, writing or physical activity. Try it. Let your emotions out—even if only a trickle.

Often in times of severe emotion (for example, during events of major destruction such as wars or bombings), people are able to think rationally and calmly and manage the acute situation well, but the underlying emotion it brings needs to be released at some point. Not dealing with emotion is often a contributor to problems such as burnout or post-traumatic stress disorder.

In his book *Opening Up*, Dr. James Pennebaker described the healing that occurs when people opened up and spoke about their past experiences.

Emotions affect behaviour

Our behaviour is directed by the way we feel. If we do not understand how we feel, or how others feel, we will not be able to understand our, or their, behaviour. If we respond to a situation with the wrong emotions, our behaviour will be misdirected. Consider the irrational behaviour of two

Introduction to Emotions

supporters of opposing sporting teams who end up in a punch-up. I am sure that the violence was never intended, but under the influence of emotions, it simply exploded.

Often, we say and do regrettable things because of our emotion. In the coolness of rationality, we are often sorry and ashamed of our behaviour during the heat of emotion.

Emotions can be unpredictable

You may have heard the comment that someone 'snapped', meaning that they were doing just fine, when suddenly their behaviour altered irrationally and wildly. This type of 'final straw on the camel's back', 'midlife crisis' or 'mental breakdown' scenario is unpredictable. Something small may trigger a world of pent-up hurt and pain, and emotions may erupt with as much force as a volcano.

When it comes to the emotions of loss and bereavement, we may sometimes experience an unpredictable outpouring of emotion triggered by something small, such as a smell or a song. Our emotions are most fragile and unpredictable during bereavement and loss.

Emotions are not reality

Emotions are so powerful, and so much a part of us, that we can imagine that they are real. While they may feel real and possibly threaten us, they only exist in our minds, and we have power over them. Often, we are troubled by irrational thoughts and emotions in the wee hours of the morning. They are not real. They need to be brought into the light of day and into the light of rationality. Do not act on an emotion until you have all the facts and can base decisions on reality and not feelings alone.

We can control our emotions

From the moment we are born, we are taught to get our emotions under control. If not, we may end up being savage, animalistic creatures, and it is the ability to control our emotions that makes us civilised. The concepts of how we control emotion are based in culture, but invariably, we all learn to not behave as a two-year-old with a temper tantrum.

We don't have to be slaves to our emotions. We can learn to sidestep less welcome emotions—we don't have to embrace every emotion.

Emotions can cause pain

As part of my palliative care training, I had the privilege of attending a lecture by Professor Ilora Finlay. She spoke about the concept of total pain, which includes physical, emotional and spiritual pain. Emotional pain is a real thing, and it can be unbearable.

She recalled a story of a patient who had uncontrollable pain. Nothing seemed to work. The patient was either 'doped out' on pain medication, or she was crying out in anguish. Her suffering was apparent. On the way home from attending a formal function in London, still dressed in her ball gown, Professor Finlay decided to go and see this patient. She sat alone with this patient in the dark room and over time realised that the lady was not suffering from physical pain but emotional pain. The thought of dying and leaving her children behind was too much for the patient to bear. The answer was not more morphine, but rather addressing this emotional distress. The breakthrough was recognising the emotional pain and treating it appropriately.

Emotions can be triggered

If you want to see me in a bad mood, put me in an airport or a queue. I am not sure why these things trigger me, but they do. I am able to realise that my behaviour is irrational when I am in a queue, and that I have to work against the frustration I feel when I am queuing.

I know what annoys me, so I can adjust my behaviour. What triggers you? Is it when the milk is left out of the fridge or when the toilet seat is not left down, or when someone is late for an appointment? Getting frustrated is not wrong, but letting your frustration boil over is not necessary. You can see it coming a hundred miles away, so why not take evasive action when you are triggered by circumstances?

Emotions have names

It is easy to think of emotions in fluffy terms, and consider them as just feelings. If we want to deal with our emotions, we will have to be honest and name them. Vague concepts like "I am feeling angry" need to be owned and condensed into "I feel angry" or "I am angry."

Once we admit to and own the emotion, we can deal with it. In dying there are many emotions to consider. Among these are fear, guilt, anger, depression, bargaining, hope, peace and love. These emotions are made real when we name them, and when we do, we can recognise each emotion for what it is, and what it is not.

Let's start with the emotion of fear.

Chapter 10

Fear, Anxiety & Worry

I often hear people say that they are not afraid of dying, and I can't help thinking that they either do not understand dying or may simply be lying. When it comes to dying, there are many, many uncertainties and unknowns. Even if life is an unbearable burden, there is always an element of uncertainty when we die, because we have not experienced it before. What if I was wrong? What if it is different to what I thought it would be? What if I forgot about something?

If you think back to your first day at school, your first ride in a roller-coaster, or your first day in a new job, you may recall the dryness of your mouth, your sweaty palms, excessive yawning, the sense of dread and palpitations, and how you wished you could be somewhere else. Thinking back, it took me far longer to get out of the car and walk into the new office environment than it normally would. Fear is not something we always think about, but it is a common emotion.

The thing about fear is that there are three versions, and often we don't separate them out enough to know the good from the bad. There is a good fear that makes us stronger and protects us from harm. It keeps us alive.

On a basic psychological level, this protective fear is the response to a direct threat. When we are directly threatened, our physiological response is to release a surge of the hormone adrenalin. This hormone primes us for action. Our heart beats faster and stronger, our pupils dilate to let in more light, our hearing improves, and our muscle tone increases. Blood is forced away from our intestines and 'lazy' organs to the muscles so they are ready for action. We become desensitised to pain, and we breathe deeply to have more oxygen available. We are prepared to escape and get away from the danger zone.

It is this surge of adrenalin that enables us to move cars and helicopters, leap over tall fences or run faster than we can imagine. This fear response to a direct threat is our unexpected friend in times of trouble. It has saved us on more than one occasion. As much as it is explosive, it is not necessarily distressing, and in small doses, this adrenaline rush can be fun.

The buzz we get from this response is why we do reckless and dangerous things, such as bungee jumping, public speaking or horse riding. If, like me, you ride horses, you'll agree that it is often an excessively adrenalin-packed adventure—for both the rider and horse—as both of us are trying to escape in different directions. This good fear has entertainment value. It is fun, especially for the spectators.

But not all fear is good. There are still two other fear types that need to be considered, and they are distressing and cause us harm. These fears are not related to a direct threat, they live in our minds, and are known as anxiety and its baby brother, worry. Both anxiety and worry are normal responses to an imagined threat. We all experience anxiety and worry, and if they remain in their cage, that is okay. But, if they are let loose, these two imagined fears can cause havoc.

Worry is a poorly defined fear that is not really connected with anything specific. It is more a sense of unfinished business and a feeling of disquiet about something that is uncertain. Worry is what keeps us awake at night. It is the attempt by our brain to identify and tie down that uncertainty. Everyone worries about death and dying at some point because of the uncertainty associated with both. Examples of things we may worry about might include:

- will I be in hospital or at home when I die?
- will I drop dead in a shopping centre or at the movies?
- will I be alone?
- will my partner and kids be okay?
- what will happen to my pets?
- who will sell the house?
- what will become of my garden?

- what happens after death?
- what if there is a God?
- what if there is no God?

These are reasonable, intangible threats, and they can be managed by rationalisation, planned actions, checklists and talking to the people who might have the answers. Trying to help the brain tie down the uncertainty will always diminish worry. The best way to stop worrying about an exam is to study. The best way to stop worrying about whether the front door is locked or not is to go and check it. If we find certainty about something, our worries will diminish. Obviously, some things cannot be resolved, and worry will stick around. Sometimes we just have to accept this and, in accepting it, put the worry on our to-do list for later and get on with what we can do now.

Unlike worry, which just lingers around like a bad smell, anxiety can be a real problem. Anxiety lives in our minds, but is not useful and, if not kept in check, it can be very harmful. The best example of the effect of anxiety allowed to get out of control is a phobia.

Perhaps the best way to understand fear, anxiety and worry is to see them in action. Imagine being invited on a fishing trip. You are not confident on boats, and you don't know much about fishing. There are a few things that worry you: will you be able to see the shore, will there be life jackets and, most importantly, will there be enough food and drink on the boat? These are normal worries, and they are resolved when you find out you can see the shore from the boat, that it is loaded with snug-fitting life jackets, and that everyone, just like you, did bring some food. See, there was nothing to worry about after all!

You are having fun, and all your worries have evaporated, when you notice a fin in the water that is unmistakably that of a big shark. Attracted by the fish and bait, it has come to have a look. As you lean over the side of the boat to have a better look at the enormous shark, your friend inadvertently bumps into you, and with a splash, you end up in the water.

At that moment your fight-or-flight survival instinct kicks in and you scream, "Shark!" In a matter of seconds, you've managed to swim back to the boat and lifted yourself back in—ignoring all the obstacles in the way. Saved by the surge of adrenalin, you are safe. Fear has served its purpose. Being afraid of a big shark in the water was a valid reaction to a real threat and triggered a response that meant you survived. You have just experienced the place of good fear in the human survival mechanism.

In contrast to this healthy fear, if you were suffering from galeophobia (an abnormal fear or anxiety about sharks), it would stop you being on the boat or anywhere even near the water. Your anxiety would have prevented you from heading out and having fun, even if there was no real threat of encountering a shark. Some people with galeophobia are so afraid that they won't even shower. Their imagined fear is that a shark could swim up the drainpipe and have a go at them. To people with this phobia, this fear is just as powerful as it would be if the threat was actually real.

As much as we may feel scorn for this extreme example, it does illustrate the evils of anxiety. Anxiety is based on a fear that exists in our imagination, rather than one that exists in the real world, and somewhere in our mind we may find the original trigger for our anxiety. When we identify the root of our anxiety, we can often regain control of it.

We all have experienced anxiety at some stage. How do you feel about public speaking? Does it cause you to feel anxious? Does your mouth go dry, and do your palms feel sweaty at the thought of speaking in front of a crowd? Public speaking is an extremely common fear, yet I know of no one who has died from it. What about the fear of spiders or cockroaches?

Anxiety is real and tangible, even though it is based on an imagined threat. It is powerful, and it affects behaviour. People will go to extremes to avoid their phobias and anxieties. They will climb twenty flights of stairs rather than get in a lift. They will make themselves ill to avoid public speaking. They will decide not to apply for a job, so they won't have to face going for an interview.

If left unchecked, anxiety may proliferate, so it is important to recognise the signs of unhealthy anxiety and get help if things seem in danger of getting out of control. If dying has you scared, and you can't stop worrying that you will turn into a zombie after you die and will come back to eat the grandkids, then there is clearly a problem.

When we break down the nature of our fears, we can recognise how they affect our lives. Telling ourselves "I am not afraid" is not really the answer to fear. We all have experienced fear in our lives, whatever its form, and we know what it is like. It is not possible to be completely without fear. The real issue is not being fearless, but being courageous and facing that fear.

We need courage in this journey at the end of life. Courage can only exist in the presence of fear, but it is greater than fear. We need courage to face the inevitable loss associated with dying, courage to dampen down the wild worries that keep us awake at night, courage to do the things that must be done, and most importantly, courage to seek help when we need it. No one is without a vulnerable spot. We are all fragile when we are exposed and feel pain.

Identifying that we are all vulnerable and admitting that this includes you, is a BIG step forward because it takes the pressure off us. We don't have to be superheroes. We can be afraid, and once we recognise that we are afraid, we have the opportunity for courage.

We all need a little help sometimes. We will talk about emotional responsibility later but, for now, if you are overcome with fear and anxiety, there is light at the end of the tunnel. Don't do it tough all on your own. Help is available. Exposing our fears and emotions makes us stronger, not weaker. It takes courage to turn on the light.

Chapter 11

Loss & Grief

In her ground-breaking 1969 work *On Death and Dying*, Elizabeth Kübler-Ross gave us permission to talk about death and dying and the emotions and feelings that follow. Prior to this, death and dying were considered taboo subjects.

What she showed us was that in dying, patients can experience a range of emotions in response to loss. Death is the ultimate loss, and depending on the extent of that loss, there is an associated outpouring of emotion. If asked, I think most people would think of loss and grief as someone sobbing or crying, perhaps inconsolably, but this is only one aspect of these emotions.

Grief does not just mean a single thing. It is the way we respond to loss. It is a complex collection of changing emotions, like a river flowing downstream. There are rapids and deadly plunging waterfalls along the way to the quiet and calm lagoon at the edge of the ocean. Knowing that grief is dynamic and changing means that we need to adapt to keep up. Elizabeth Kübler-Ross described five stages of emotion in response to loss: shock and denial, anger, depression, bargaining and, finally, acceptance.

The emotional responses to loss can be varied. People do not necessarily experience all these emotions. They do not necessarily all come in order, and some people may have an entirely different emotional response to loss. These emotions are not linear like a ruler with a point A and B. They are more like a coiled ball of string with many touch points and loops backwards and forwards. These emotions can come and go, and come again. As with all emotions, it may be messy. Elizabeth Kübler-Ross's stage model of grief has recognised flaws, but it is a great starting point to recognise a normal response to loss and realise that it is perfectly normal to feel loss.

These emotions of grief are not only limited to the loss associated with dying. They can also be part of any loss, such as a lost relationship, a lost promotion, or when your favourite team loses in the final.

We have all experienced loss, and we may recognise our own emotional response when it occurs. If not, consider the example of little Lucy, a two-year-old child on a shopping expedition with her mum. She wants an ice cream *now*, but her request is denied: "No!" Her first response is a sense of incredulity and shock. She cannot believe that her request has been denied. This shock phase does not last long, and it is almost immediately followed by the anger phase. Lucy goes limp and falls on the floor, throwing a massive temper tantrum—kicking and screaming on the ground. This does not produce an ice cream, so depression sets in, and Lucy starts to cry inconsolably for a few minutes before she realises this won't succeed either. She then starts bargaining, asking for a lolly instead of an ice cream.

After the ongoing rejection of her demands, she resigns herself to the fact that she will not get an ice cream, and the shopping expedition continues peacefully until the next shopping aisle where she sees a soft fluffy rabbit and wants it. We know how the story unfolds from here. Shopping with a two-year-old is a hazard, and it requires master level psychology skills to survive.

If you think about the losses you've experienced in your life, you will recognise some of these emotions. They are there if we care to look. Remember that flat tyre you had last year? Chances are you were shocked at the discovery of a flat, kicked the tyre in frustration, angrily changed the tyre, felt down about it for the day and then moved on. Or if you think about that one promotion you did not get—the shock, then the anger, then the bargaining (even if it is only in your mind), the dreams of other employment and, finally, accepting the loss and carrying on. I speak from experience. Loss is not fun, and the emotions are often more than we expect.

During the experience of a loss associated with a terminal illness, all these emotions are possible and probable. The intensity of the emotions experienced can be as uninhibited as a two-year-old's tantrum. These emotions are very real, they can change without warning, and they can be harmful if we do not deal with them appropriately.

Being emotionally aware and recognising these normal emotions allows us to manage them before they spin out of control and cause damage.

In my work, I have had to sit quietly and simply be there for patients or their relatives who break down at the shock news of incurable cancer and a limited prognosis. The shock brings a numbness, and in my experience, it is like you suddenly have tunnel vision, but with all your other senses, too. When my brother-in-law was diagnosed with advanced pancreatic cancer, I received the news as I was driving my son to school. In shock, I was unaware of my speed until I was pulled over by the police. I was not even able to adequately defend myself. I was only able to mumble apologies and I drove off with a fine and a handful of demerit points.

We advise and train our staff not to push back at patients or carers who are in the anger phase of loss. Knowing how likely it is that they will be feeling angry, we give them space to vent. Knowing some will be feeling sad and depressed, we allow them to experience this normal emotion of loss and work their way through it. It is not always necessary to intervene if there is a normal emotional reaction playing out. We will discuss anger and depression later because they are so important.

Bargaining gives one thing in the hope of being able to take another back. This is where those undergoing loss try to find an alternative truth, or at least, a reprieve from the loss. They will often pay anything for a small win.

When it comes to the bargaining phase of grief, it is nice to be on the receiving end. In our department, this is when patients will bring us gifts of chocolate and flowers, in the hope that we can make things better. Perhaps, we can make them live longer? Perhaps if they are nice to us, we can keep the cancer away, or we will give them better treatment? Who can resist a good bargain?

- If I say my prayers, and go to church again, then perhaps God will heal me?
- If I can't be cured, then perhaps I can live another 24 months?
- If I bake cookies for the oncology unit perhaps they will treat me better and I will live longer?

Mrs Shaefer was a memorable patient who maximised the benefits of bargaining for all the oncologists along the coast. She had been diagnosed with incurable Stage 4 breast cancer. Although she was not yet close to death, there was no prospect of a cure. With this background she would go and see an oncologist bearing gifts and kind words—sparing no expense. The whiskey, for those who enjoyed it, was top shelf.

She came bearing gifts when she came to see me. She was seeking a second opinion, and I'd ended up number two on what would eventually become a long list of oncologists she would consult in her quest to be healed. I listened as she told me all about how terrible the previous oncologist was, and how she had total and complete trust in me. She preened my ego and made me feel successful and accomplished—welcome flattery for a young and inexperienced oncologist.

I did my best to treat her, but as with all the other doctors she saw, I couldn't offer her the cure that she wanted. So, she abandoned me. I found out later from a close oncologist friend that she then went to see him bearing gifts, telling him what a terrible oncologist I was and ensuring his ego was equally well massaged. He could not heal her either, so he also rapidly became part of the flotsam and jetsam of oncologists left in her wake.

The bargaining phase is the riskiest for those going through loss. For them, any win is welcome, and it is here where the charlatans of care make their profits. It is here the unproven 'cures' are attractive, and people will pay vast fortunes for these unachievable promises.

- No, photodynamic light therapy at a Centre of Excellence in Mexico is not going to cure your daughter of Stage 4 cancer, sorry.
- No, magnet therapy in Germany is not going to save your life if your time has come, sorry!

The lines between bargaining and denial may sometimes seem blurred. With denial there is no room for any failure, but with bargaining it is the opposite, there is hope for a win. Bargaining is hopeful against the odds. If your football team is 4–0 down, five minutes before the end of the game, bargaining will convince you it is not over yet. There is a small chance for a win, perhaps even a miracle!

Finally, the whistle blows. The results are up and the final score line isn't going to change. The game is over. There is no chance of wining. It is time to accept that your team has lost, and move on to face the reality of the situation. This does not need to be a depressing or sad moment. This is a good moment because now you stop holding your breath waiting for the impossible. Now, you can get on with your life again!

The final stage of loss is acceptance, where the night passes away and the sun rises on a new day of opportunity. This is where you get your life back, even if it is a short one. This is where you get permission to move on and do the things YOU want to do, rather than the things dictated to you by disease and illness and hospitals and doctors. Once you have accepted the loss associated with death and dying, it can no longer hurt you. You may experience the inconvenience of physical symptoms and the normal wild emotions and the questions that remain, but in this space, *you* now get to choose how you live the rest of your life.

Knowing and recognising the stages of loss allows us to do damage control. The problem is that often we only focus on the person dying and forget to look around. Their spouses, friends, family, children and grandchildren may also all be feeling loss, and sometimes this loss is greater than the one experienced by the person dying. Those who are spectators may also experience shock, anger and depression. They may also push the barrow of bargaining and insist on unproven remedies found down uncertain avenues.

My hope is that we can all eventually come to the stage of acceptance. But this is an unrealistic and unkind expectation for some people. It is not always possible to move from one base to the next. Not everyone experiences all (or any) of these emotions. Chances are that people will respond to loss as they have with all the other losses in their life. This may be with humour, or they may simply face facts and get on with life.

There is no right or wrong when it comes to grief, apart from recognising that it is at play and allowing it time to resolve. People in grief do not always need counselling, hugs or "Are you OK?" affirmations. Sometimes all they need is space and time, and perhaps a cup of tea at the right time.

Chapter 12

Anger

Anger is a fantastic emotion. If you want to get attention and get what you want, get angry! This is something we learn early in life and, unless we have been taught to be civilised and kind, our anger can be a powerful weapon, and a means of getting our own way.

Fortunately, anger is frowned upon in society, otherwise we would all be slamming doors, pounding desks and shouting obscenities, all the time. We don't tolerate anger—we feel uncomfortable with it.

As spectators, our usual response to anger is either to run away from it or to respond in kind. We don't often stop to examine this explosive and destructive emotion. When we do, it is best done with caution and from a distance.

Anger can manifest in a number of ways. The first type of anger is spontaneous, explosive anger, as seen in road rage incidences. If you are bored and have nothing better to do, search for road rage on YouTube. In the wrong set of circumstances, perfectly normal people who probably eat cornflakes for breakfast and who have kids and well-paying jobs, lose it and become monsters. They do things they would never have planned or contemplated in a million years.

What sets off this behaviour? There can be many triggers for anger. Failed expectations can be a trigger for loss, and anger is one of the powerful emotions we have to endure as we come to terms with it. Other causes can include being late for a meeting, getting stuck in gridlocked traffic, not knowing the answers to a quiz or being forced to listen to a long, recorded message when you need to speak to someone on the phone urgently.

Our behaviour when angry can often be regrettable. We may call someone an "old cow" or punch the wall, or if we are at home, hurt the feelings of those we love the most. Sometimes, we cannot solve the unsolvable problem. By accepting this, and realising that traffic is traffic, exam quizzes are sometimes difficult, and the call to the government department can wait, we no longer need anger as a response. Does anger change the unsolvable situation or make it better? No. Anger has no purpose other than letting off steam. It is an important valve to release pressure, but anger is seldom the solution to anything.

The second type of anger is not just an expression of deep frustration but has also become a behaviour choice. Some people use anger as a tool. They know that getting angry gets results, and it works. If you are angry and abusive, shouting at the staff in any situation, chances are they will respond quickly and get you what you want because no one wants to contend with an angry person.

Angry people are always the ones who get attention. They don't make any friends, but they do get their voice heard. Often it is a good strategy to make some noise and be that irritating person. It's the person yelling about the long lines on a busy day who is given the next medical appointment ahead of a queue of waiting people. Meek and mild older people waiting patiently and being polite will always come second. There is no fairness when you use anger to your benefit.

We have all experienced hot anger: shouting, cursing, door slamming, wall punching. It is threatening to be around, and unless you are up for a fight and willing to show some aggression, most of us will concede and make way for an angry person. You need to be brave (or stupid) to get in the way, and if you do, it is often also out of anger. It is easy to recognise the signs of explosive anger and to get out of the way and seek shelter.

Anger, however, is not always hot and explosive. It can be equally destructive when served cold. This third type of anger is not clearly demonstrated, but it is distinctly felt. Here there is no clear demonstration of feelings, but rather an icy response to anything that gets in the way. It is the silent assassin out to get revenge and inflict pain. It is the cold shoulder; the silent treatment you get for a misdemeanour or minor offense, and unlike explosive anger, it can endure until revenge has been fully satisfied.

- This is the person who says, "Yes, dear," and you know very well it is a harbinger of trouble, and that apologies are urgently required.
- This is the person who smiles at you as they lodge a complaint against you.
- This is the person who greets you with a hug, only to plunge the dagger in your back.

I would love to say this is not me. That I don't get angry. That I am not explosive. That I do not demand to have it my way. That I am not an icy, angry person. But that would not be true. Given the right circumstances, I can get very angry.

Anger is a normal emotion. We all get angry at some time, one way or another. There's no perfect state of zen where we can always simply switch off our feelings. What triggers your anger?

- Seeing a child being abused?
- Seeing an animal being abused?
- A bully at work?
- Being ill and not being able to do anything about it?
- Having to pay medical bills?
- Not being served to your expectation in a restaurant?

Not all anger is bad, and it is not always wrong to be angry. Sometimes we do need to get angry and direct that anger towards achieving justice. Seeing a child abused or someone bullied at work requires the anger to put a stop to it. Being denied medical care for a loved one requires an anger that won't give up trying until they get it. Mediocrity and slackness need to receive an angry reception that will be a motivation to make sure it isn't repeated.

However, it is important to stop and consider the consequences. Is getting angry going to achieve anything or make things any better? If you are angry with your doctor and handle it badly, will it compromise future care? It may!

We cannot always undo the damage we do in anger. Rage and murder are one thing, but sometimes, it is the subtle harm we do with our angry words that causes the greatest harm:

- You are so stupid!
- You say the dumbest things!
- I wish I never met you!
- It's fine for you to be cheerful and happy, you're not the one dying.
- You'll probably find a new wife as soon as I am gone.
- You don't really care about me. You can't wait for me to die!
- I wish you would just get it over with and die.
- I wish you had cancer like me.

Because we can hurt people in the heat of anger, it is worth having a cooling down strategy. Being 'anger aware' is a good skill to have. A hot-headed decision is never going to be the best, so defer making one until the anger has passed. It always does. Cold anger requires a different strategy: grace and forgiveness. It is not useful to be angry with someone forever, because forever is a very long time.

If anger is causing your relationships to fail, please consider an anger management strategy. If necessary, get professional help. Find a way to keep the fuse burning for longer before you explode, avoid situations that are potentially explosive, and when you can, be gracious. We all make mistakes, and if you have been wrongfully treated, consider letting it go. It is not worth holding the hot coals of anger in your hand forever. It is not worth the effort of maintaining a cold anger once the moment has passed. Let it go and move on, not for the sake of the offender but for yourself.

Chapter 13

Depression & Sadness In Loss

Depression and sadness are emotions that come with loss. We have all experienced this response to loss at some stage. It may have been the death of a grandparent or parent. It may have been the death of a pet, or the death of a relationship, or the 'death' of employment opportunity. Regardless of the nature of the loss, the emotional response of sadness or depression often comes with tears. In the era in which I grew up, tears were often considered a sign of weakness, and we were told, "Boys don't cry." But tears signify we are hurting and vulnerable, so we need to talk about tears and what they mean.

We cry for several reasons, ranging from chopping onions to experiencing strong feelings associated with beauty or as a response to love, frustration, anger, sadness or loss. We are the only species of animal that cry. Tears are a signal of our vulnerability, reflecting what is going on in our hearts. Big, burly blokes cry at their daughters' weddings, whereas some people do not cry at all.

Physiologically, there is no clear benefit to crying, so why do we cry at all? It was once thought that tears originated from the heart, but we now know that they do not, at least from a physiological perspective. Tears come from the tear glands on the upper outer side of each eye. Running along the tear duct, they lubricate the eye before draining into the nose. That is why we get a runny nose when we cry, and why, when we sob, there is a hideous mess of tears and snot and tissues.

In the 1600s, people believed that strong emotions, especially love, heated the heart, and produced 'heart vapour' that rose to the head and escaped as tears. I think they were onto something. Where do the feelings that cause tears originate from? I think that they do come from the heart, the centre of our emotion. Neuroscience tells us emotions are chemical signals in the brain, but those of us who have recently wept know they come from the heart. That is where we hurt when we cry, and it is where it hurts that makes us cry.

When last did you cry? Was it triggered by a powerful emotion? How did you feel when you cried? Was that feeling in your heart or was it in your mind? Regardless of the cause, nature or purpose of tears, they are a great emotional release valve, and in the long run, they do us good.

In dying, the loss we feel is so great that there are many

reasons to cry. We have to say goodbye to and let go of so many things we value. We have to say goodbye to ourselves, to our lives, to the things that defined us, to our careers and to the things that give us meaning. We have to say goodbye to those we dearly love: husbands and wives, children, grandchildren, lifetime friends. For some, saying goodbye to their pet dog or cat is unbearably difficult.

In dying, our goodbyes include the things we love and enjoy doing. We have to say goodbye to the things of this world: the embrace of our loved ones, the moments with grandkids, the walks on the beach, the whistling for the dog to fetch the ball, the smell of baking, the taste of a fig jam. They will all be coming to an end. Our hearts ache, and we are allowed to cry.

We might cry in the privacy of our own space when we are alone. We might cry unexpectedly, triggered by a memory or a smell or a sound. We might cry softly lying in bed in the early hours of the morning. We might cry in each other's arms. All these are manifestations of sadness.

Sadness is a normal feeling. It is unpleasant in nature, and it is unpredictable. Sadness interrupts a normal day, while we are having normal thoughts and feelings. It can unexpectedly pop up in a happy moment. Sadness sneaks up on us and may leave as quickly as it comes. That's the key. Unlike depression, sadness comes and goes, and it does not last long. It requires no intervention. It is normal to feel sad and we need to allow sadness the time to work its way through our current and future loss.

Sadness becomes a problem when it sticks around until there are no longer any happy days. When this happens, we are possibly dealing with depression, and this is a tough ride. To meet the definition of depression, someone must feel depressed for more than two weeks. Their feelings of depression must affect their ability to function in society, and these feelings must not be associated with illness or medication.

These requirements for a diagnosis of depression are very similar to the symptoms exhibited by someone who is dying, and this can make the diagnosis of depression difficult. Often the illness, pain, and morphine all contribute to a patient feeling down. And trying to separate a diagnosis of depression out of this complex situation is difficult.

Depression is characterised by a low mood or diminished interest in activities or pleasure. It is a bleak place to be, and where sadness blames its cause, depression blames the self. In depression, there are feelings of worthlessness and poor self-esteem.

Haven't we all at some point felt too sad to be able to do anything other than sit in our room and do nothing for a few hours or a day or two? When this feeling occurs day after day, and there is no joy or happiness—or even the anticipation of happiness—it is time to go see the doctor and get some help. Depression is a weight too heavy to carry on your own.

When we defined death, we said it was the absence of a response to stimulus. In the same way, depression is an 'emotional death'. There is less and less response to emotional stimulus, until there is no response at all. If you or someone you know is dying emotionally, please get help.

Our emotions change, and the emotion of sadness will also come and go. Being sad is okay. Recognising emotions as a normal response to loss is important because it gives us permission to feel them and work through them. Being aware of depression in others or ourselves allows us to ask for help, and we all sometimes need help.

But not every tear needs a tissue, and not every lonely moment needs to be rescued. Mourning the approach of death is normal. You don't have to 'cheer up', and those who suggest this as a solution for depression or sadness need to spend some time in the stocks. I will bring the rotten tomatoes.

It is in this time of tears that we need to accept that we are vulnerable. It is good to express our sadness, and it is good to let it out. Tears make us human.

Chapter 14

Guilt & Regret

Wouldn't it be wonderful to have a time machine and be able to go back in time? It would be great to relive some of those amazing moments in our lives—the ones we wish could have gone on and on. Like the time we had our first kiss, or when we graduated from school never to go back, or the birth of our children and grandchildren. There are so many good memories that the time machine would be flat out dashing back to all these wonderful experiences. But then, we would probably not have time to do anything else.

Not all of our past is wonderful. There are things that have happened in our lives that we regret. If we could get into the time machine, many of us would be visiting the times we messed things up. We would seize missed opportunities. We would take back hurtful words, and we would undo unforgivable actions. But, because this wonderful time machine does not exist, we are stuck with these bad decisions and actions.

While poor decisions may not bother us in the hustle and bustle of daily life, they can become an issue when we have too much time to think and realise that there are not going to be any second chances. Many people struggle with regret and guilt when life is ending. These emotions of regret and guilt differ. They need to be put into perspective because, when it comes to dying, they should not be on the invitation list.

The emotion of regret

Regret is a feeling of sadness or disappointment associated with failure. We have all failed to some degree in life, but while we all have regrets, not all these regrets are valid. Some regrets may be short-lived, as in, "I wish I had not had that third helping of dessert" or "I wish I *did* have a helping of dessert" when you missed it. Other failures can follow us all our life. No one is perfect, and the opportunities for failure and regret in life are boundless.

Sometimes we regret what life has done to us. Things do not always work out the way we think they should have, and this can leave us feeling short-changed, particularly when we realise that our dreams are never going to be realised. Some of these regrets should not be valid because they were not under our control. It is as if an invisible hand has reached out and prevented us from doing what we set out to achieve, and as a result our lives have turned out differently to what we had imagined.

- Perhaps you never managed to get into the medical training program to be a doctor.
- Perhaps you did not make the grade to be a police officer.
- Perhaps you did not marry the person of your dreams.
- Perhaps your desire to be a farmer never eventuated.
- Perhaps you never managed to become a millionaire.

We do not always understand why these things didn't happen for us. It is not for lack of trying!

We don't get to see the big picture, but if we could, we might be surprised to find that being a doctor is not the greatest job ever, that police officers get injured, that the person of your dreams turned out to be an abusive psychopath, that farmers were subject to record-breaking droughts and that a million bucks would never be enough because you would want to have a billion.

Looking back and thinking about the opportunities that passed by and what might have been when the road ahead is short and uncertain is a tempting form of self-harm. If your life did not turn out the way you expected due to circumstances outside of your control, how can you be held responsible? If you are still holding onto past dreams that were never meant to be more than a dream, let them go.

Guilt

We have a handle on most emotions, and we can control them, but guilt is an emotion that controls us. The more we try to compensate for guilt, the worse it becomes. It is a shady character preferring to lurk in darkness. Once it is exposed to light, it is gone.

Unlike regret that is not related to wrongdoing, guilt is spawned out of wrongdoing. Guilt is a feeling of regret or shame over having done something wrong. If we are unaware of our offense or don't care, or if we don't think we have done anything wrong, we will not feel guilty. It is only when we have done something wrong or believe that we have done something wrong that we feel guilty.

Guilt sticks out, and it is eventually visible to all. My mum, and I'm sure yours as well, knew when I had done something wrong. It may have been when I stole the neighbour's oranges, when I did not do my homework, or when I told a lie. How on earth did she know? It is because guilt changes our behaviour. When we feel guilty, our behaviour may change to include:

- overcompensation—we try too hard to get everything right
- oversensitivity and defensive behaviour about doing anything wrong
- denial—rationalising and pretending nothing is wrong
- inflicting ongoing punishment on others who are guilty of doing something wrong.

When we have done something wrong, we cover it up with these behavioural changes. We may think we have beaten the system, but nobody is buying it. No one can act so perfect all the time, no one should be so defensive, no one can be so rational about everything and no one should be so eager to mete out punishment. The change in our normal behaviour is soon so apparent that even our parents, and anyone else who is looking, know we are guilty about something.

These behavioural changes are obstacles to normal relationships. They get in the way, and they trip us up. We don't intend to feel guilty. It is not an emotion we can manage. It is simply there.

There are two types of guilt, and it is important to distinguish them. The first is when we think or believe we have done, (or are doing) something wrong, but we have not (or are not). This is common when it comes to dying. Those who are going to carry on living feel guilty about it and it changes their behaviour. They feel guilty about not being able to fix an unfixable problem. They feel guilty of their good fortune.

- I will be here to enjoy life, but Harry won't.
- It is my fault Donna did not stop smoking.
- I am so tired I wish this was all just over.
- Mary is dying and she won't get to see the grandkids, but I will.

- I wish David would just die. I just can't do this anymore.
- It should be me instead of Rose who is dying.

Similarly, those who are dying may feel the same guilt. They feel they are doing something wrong in dying and they may feel guilty that they won't be there to fulfil their role. They may believe that their dying and its consequences are selfish acts.

- I won't be there to mow the lawn.
- Who is going to take care of Anne?
- I won't be able to attend the board meeting.
- I won't be able to make it to Sophie's wedding.

For both parties, guilt is misdirected because no one has done anything wrong. Unless you are God and have power over life and death, there is nothing you can do about being mortal. It is not your fault if a life is ending. It is not wrong to die. It is the journey we must all undertake, and if you think that it is evil to die, think again. This guilt is an imposter and the easiest way around it is to talk about it and bring it into the light. Don't accept responsibility for something you have not done. Don't accept guilt, no matter who wants to give it to you or how attractive the packaging may seem. Being blamed for something you have not done is not fair to you. If you have guilt and it doesn't fit, don't wear it.

The second type of guilt *does* fit, and it is due to having done (or doing) something wrong. This guilt is associated with the mistakes we make in life. Can we fix it? Of course, we can.

The first thing to do is to stop doing what is wrong. The second is to admit to the wrongdoing. It is a behavioural response to the wrongness we don't want exposed. When you are busted, you no longer feel guilty—you *are* guilty. For many, this brings a sense of relief. In James Pennebaker's book *Opening up*, he explains that confession is healthy. We cannot always fix all the things we have done wrong in our life, but we can get rid of the burden of guilt when we bring the wrongdoing into the light.

But this needs wisdom. Don't confess publicly if your confession is going to do more harm than good. Don't confess to being Suzie's father if Suzie and her family are living happy fulfilled lives, blissfully unaware of this truth. Don't tell your wife about the secret affair with your secretary thirty years ago if it is not going to be fixable. Not all wrongs need to be brought into the public light and made right in front of everyone's eyes. Wisdom recognises that time may have healed over the wounds of past transgressions and opening them up will just hurt people and not help anyone. Sometimes, there is nothing more that needs to be said or done about a matter.

If you are guilty, the third thing to do, the bonus option, is to seek is forgiveness. This is not always possible.

It may not always be available, or it may not be given by the one who has been harmed. Sorry is a powerful word. If you are not sure, give it a try. Sometimes the only person we need to forgive is ourselves and if the shoe fits, there is forgiveness and redemption with God for those who seek it.

Chapter 15

Emotional Responsibility

When we are dying everything is going wrong. In other activities, like learning to play tennis or perfecting a golf swing, things get better with practice. In dying things only get worse. Easy things we may have taken for granted, like walking up a flight of stairs or driving the car, are no longer an option. As the body fails and more things go wrong, frustration, impatience and anger are not uncommon. Emotions run high—everyone is fatigued, everyone is just sick of it all!

The emotions of loss are ever-present, and with each new loss there is a risk of repeating the whole emotional cycle all over again. Those who are spectators also feel the loss, and they are primed for an explosive emotional outburst. We can see a powder keg of emotion ready to explode, and because of this, we need to have some emotional responsibility and risk management. It is worth having a game plan if you don't want to be blown up. My father taught me that *a* plan is better than no plan.

Following are some survival strategies, and I am sure you will discover your own ones that work best for you:

Accept that 'it is what it is'

We all have a breaking point and to expect anything less will break you. Fatigue, pain, uncertainty, financial distress and a life filled with medical appointments all add to the burden of illness. While we may survive an assault on one front, often multiple assaults on every front will overwhelm us. Feeling emotionally overwhelmed is not unusual.

In his book *Good to Great*, Jim Collins tells a story about Vice Admiral James Stockdale in which he describes the Stockdale Paradox. On 9 September 1965, then-Commander Stockdale was shot down over enemy territory in Vietnam and held as a prisoner of war at the infamous 'Hanoi Hilton'. Against remarkable odds, and after enduring terrible torture, he survived. The reason was that he was willing to face the facts and brutal reality of his situation. He accepted that he had to go through the trials and not around them.

There are some brutal facts about dying, and if you want to prepare for it properly, it is important to accept these facts and deal with them. Dying is something we will all have to 'go through' not 'go around'. Knowledge makes this possible. In Julius Caesar, Shakespeare wrote:

> A coward dies a thousand times before his death, but the valiant taste of death but once. It seems to me most strange that men should fear, seeing that death, a necessary end, will come when it will come.

Emotions are not reality

In Chapter 10, we discussed the nature of emotions. As much as they can be powerful, they don't endure. They are not always based on fact, and they can change if we give them permission to change.

We may feel angry right now, but if we just wait our anger may subside. We may feel depressed and down in the dumps right now, but tomorrow is a new day and we may feel different. Knowing that emotions are variable allows us the opportunity to 'not get on the bus' of a bad emotion, but to let it pass and wait for the next bus of a better emotion to come long.

Have a game plan

When the fighter jet has been hit and is going down, it is handy to have an 'ejection seat'. When the proverbial crap is hitting the fan, don't just stand there—get out of the way. Have an escape route. Stomping your foot harder or longer in frustration is not a good way to manage an unfixable situation. Have a strategy.

- Go for a walk when you are feeling strong emotions.
- Take your mind off the problem for a while: read a book, play a game, watch telly, write your story.
- Pick your moments—my wife and I never discuss anything important after 10 pm as we recognise that we are both tired by then, and any conflict

situation is bound to be more explosive.
- Know what triggers your emotions and plan for it—I hate filling in forms of any description so, as much as possible, I get someone else to do it.
- When all else fails hold your breath for a minute…See? You feel better already!

Don't do 'emotional DIY'

If you had a broken car, you would go to a mechanic. If you had an overflowing toilet, you would ask for a plumber. If your tooth was hurting you would visit a dentist, and if your arm was broken, you would see a doctor. It all makes perfect sense, until there's an emotional breakdown. When it comes to emotional issues, most of us think we can fix it by ourselves, and we end up creating a real DIY disaster in the process.

If you have an emotional problem, please see a psychologist, counsellor, social worker, priest, or at least, some sort of trained person who can help. Do not ask your plumber. You may end up with a piece of piping that does not fit. Do not ask your hairdresser, and don't ask your friends who also have no idea. Get help from the professionals.

Let your feelings out—talk and listen

Talk about your feelings, even if you are not sure how you feel. Get them out, let them be free. Let others talk about their feelings, too, and listen to what they are saying. Create a safe space where things can be said without there being drama. Find a way to let off steam safely—we all know what happens to pressure cookers when the steam cannot escape.

Sometimes, this is where professional help is needed. We don't always have to use words to talk. We can express our feelings in writing, poetry, music or art. Just let them out.

Give yourself and others a break

Sometimes I can be a real pain. I will admit it, I am known to take things too seriously, and I can curl myself into a tight little ball of responsibility. I can overanalyse what people say or pretend I know what they think.

If you find that you are getting too wound-up, give yourself a break. Have a holiday. Have a down day where, no matter what the drama is in life, you won't react or respond. It can wait until tomorrow. Have a 'be nice to yourself day' and, if possible, include those around you as well. Not all issues have to be an issue.

Know why, and when, you need to get help

Emotions can be destructive, and if left unmanaged they are going to hurt *those you love*. If we love someone, we owe it to them and ourselves to protect them and care for them. Getting emotional help when our emotions are out of control is one way we can demonstrate our love for both ourselves and those we love.

If your everyday is a conflict-filled war zone, get help.

If you are not feeling any emotion at all or if you might be depressed, get help. If you are always angry and, as a result, are destroying things, get help. If you can't cope with the bad emotions and behaviour of those you love, get help.

Sometimes, getting help is as easy as pulling a thorn out of a hurting foot—ouch, and it's over. It feels better immediately, and you wonder why you waited so long to get rid of the thorn. The word 'sorry' works a lot like that. But often, it is more complicated.

Know when there is a storm coming and be ready for it. Batten down the hatches before the storm hits. Don't be afraid to ask for directions if you feel lost.

Aim for happiness

I often remind myself and my patients that we should aim for the top of Mt Everest, but if we don't get there, then Base Camp is good enough. Sometimes, we cannot achieve what we set out to do, and that is okay, but we must still set out. There must be a goal.

One of our quests in life is for happiness. This emotion is very rare—mostly we seem to just be existing. In the chaos of life, and in dying, dare we hope for happiness? Or is this out of our reach? We don't often stop to think about being happy. Many of us may ask, "What does that even mean?"

It is hard to imagine that anyone can be happy or content against the setting of a terminal illness, yet Mrs Blades was happy. Through all that we have discussed—the pain, the frustration, the symptoms, the loss and even in the 'dying'—she was at peace; she was content. She was happy.

Look up

When it comes to dying it is easy to keep looking down into the bottomless pit of despair. There is no light or hope there. The longer you stare into it, the darker it becomes. There is another way, but it requires us to deliberately look up, away from the disaster of dying, to focus on the opportunities for living. For that we need hope.

Hope is the greatest emotion we can have when all else is failing.

Chapter 16

Faith & Hope

In 2003, Aron Ralston set off on a solo mountain climbing journey. On his way down Bluejohn Canyon, a huge boulder was dislodged, trapping his arm at the wrist. Try as he might, he could not dislodge the huge boulder or free his crushed arm. He had to endure pain and conquer his fear. He had to go through the emotional stages of loss: denial, anger, depression, bargaining and, eventually acceptance.

The facts were bleak. There was no escape and Ralston only had limited food and water remaining before he would run out. He accepted his fate of death. He recorded his final goodbyes and drank his last drop of water. Then, in a state of near hallucination, he realised that he could survive without his arm. In that instant, he had found the hope to live.

In a superhuman feat driven by hope, Ralston smashed through the bones in his forearm, then used a tourniquet and blunt multi-tool to amputate his arm. Once free, he managed to make it down the canyon where he was found and rescued.

Against all odds he had survived—he had paid a huge price, but he had survived. His story has now been dramatized in the movie *127 Hours*. His arm was also retrieved by rescuers after the massive boulder was moved. It was cremated and returned it to him at a later date. The arm was not much use to him in powder form, but I expect he appreciated the gesture. It is always better to be fully armed than unarmed.

Hope is a funny thing; it can exist in the darkest of places and shine as the brightest of lights. Hope is what sustained Aron. The amazing story of Louis Zamperini also tells of hope. He survived being shot down in World War II, spending 47 days adrift at sea before being rescued, only to suffer later in a Japanese war camp. His amazing story of survival is dramatised in the movie *Unbroken*.

In the Stockdale Paradox, the first requirement was to face the brutal facts and reality of the situation. The second part of the paradox was to maintain hope and faith in a future. On the one hand is the darkness, on the other the light. Both are required, because hope without darkness is not really hope at all. The darker it is, the more we need hope.

Hope is a feeling, or a desire, based on something that has not happened yet. Because it is looking forward to some future moment, it really has no substance—the future has not yet happened. The promise that there is a future is all hope offers.

Hope is what ultimately motivates us. It is why we get

out of bed in the morning and take the next step. Hope is always positive. If it were not for hope, we would not study for an exam, go to work, or have children. We do these things with the belief that they are worthwhile, and if things are not great now, they will be.

Without hope, we are defeated before we even start. No one should experience hopelessness. It is for those who have no future nor will ever have a future. It demeans us and forces us to exist rather than to live.

Five kinds of hope

There are five kinds of hope, all based on differing levels of probability.

First, there is the realistic hope. This is based on a high level of probability, and mostly these hopes are achievable with a little bit of planning and minimal effort. This is hope that is within our power, and we can, apart from bad luck, make it happen if we want to. These are the hopes of bucket-lists, things to do and to realistically expect.

- This is the hope to be pain free.
- This is the hope to die at home.
- This is the hope that my family can be with me when I die.
- This is the hope to find a good home for my dog.
- This is the hope to go hot air ballooning before I die.

- This is the hope to get medical care and see a palliative care physician.

The second hope is less secure and is based on a lower probability, but the outcome may still be achieved with our best efforts and a bit of luck.

- This is the hope of having chemotherapy that offers a 5% survival chance, but it is worth it.
- It is the hope of passing an exam if you have not studied for it.
- It is the hope of catching a fish.
- It is the hope held by everyone who plays golf.
- It is the hope that I can get to visit Venice before I die.

Then there is the miraculous hope. These hopes are based on a very low probability of ever happening, but the probability is still not zero. Miracles do happen. These hopes are outside of our control, yet we dare to believe in them. They make us keep going, even though they may never happen.

- I hope for a cure to this cancer.
- I hope that the new trial drug works.
- I hope to get to Christmas.
- I hope to see my birthday.
- I hope to be able to see my son get married.
- I hope for a miracle.

Wishful thinking is the fourth kind of hope. It requires no effort and no action, and it has a zero probability. Even so, it makes us feel better about our other misdirected actions. We are all guilty of it. We know it won't work, but it is worth trying because we have no options. We don't feel depressed when this hope does not eventuate because it was so unachievable, and we did not really expect it to work out in the first place, but we feel we at least tried.

- You will pass an exam, even if you never attended lectures or studied for it.
- You will be able to talk your way out of a speeding ticket.
- Requires a time-warp: if it takes 30 minutes to get to the airport and there are only 10 minutes left. This is the hope that expects to get there on time.
- The traffic lights, which always take 90 seconds to change, will change sooner if you wish hard enough.

Finally, there is false hope, which is denial in disguise. It has a zero probability of happening, but we hold onto it because we feel empowered by doing so. The harder it is, the better we feel because we are doing something, and that is better than doing nothing. The problem is that the probability is zero, and all our time and effort is wasted when we could be doing other, better things. This is the hope that believes:

- unproven treatments such as sodium bicarbonate will cure cancer
- only Dr Adam Smith, a living legend in Mexico, can cure cancer
- a sugar-free diet will cure cancer
- drinking apple cider vinegar will make you live longer.

Each one of these different kinds of hope are based on something in the future, but they require action today. If you hope to go to town, your action will be to get dressed and get in the car to go to town. If you hope to go hot air ballooning, it requires the action to phone the hot air balloon operators and book an adventure. If you hope to go swimming, the action required is finding water and, if you are inclined, wear swimming gear when you swim.

Hope motivates us. It forces us to take action. The action we take is an act of faith. A farmer has faith that the potatoes he planted will come up, so his action includes watering the potatoes. A train driver hopes to get to his destination and that the tracks will all be in working order, and when he sets off, he acts in faith that all will be well. A car driver hopes that they will get to their destination, and the action of driving is an act of faith. We all have faith as we act on our hope.

There is one hope that outshines all the other hopes in dying, and that is the hope that we are immortal. We have always held the hope that we do not have to die and taste the bitterness of death. It has been in our hearts, this hope of immortality. While this may seem to be in the category of denial or a wishful thinking kind of hope, the reality is that we have been right all along.

There is evidence to support the notion that as spiritual beings, we are immortal. Death is not the end of us, but merely the end of our physical bodies.

To understand this, we need to turn to spirituality. This is our greatest hope.

Chapter 17

Introduction To Spirituality

The ancient Greeks believed that, at the time of death, the spirit would leave the body as a little puff of breath, and Thanatos, the god of the dead, would collect the soul of the dying and carry it lovingly and kindly to the River Styx. There the soul would be handed over to Charon, the ferryman. For the correct price of coins placed on the eyes of the deceased, Charon would transfer the soul to the underworld and into the hands of Hades. Here the soul would continue to exist.

The pharaohs of ancient Egypt were so convinced about life after death, and concerned about the welfare of their souls, that they allocated vast resources to prepare for a better afterlife. There were at least 20,000 people working on the pyramids at any one time, reaching around 40,000 at peak times of the year.

These vast numbers of workers were required in order to move such an immense amount of stone. Parties of slaves would use rollers to transport 2500 kg blocks of stone during the building of the pyramids. Eighteen men could move one of these vast blocks 18 metres in a minute. It is quite amazing that they still had a workforce after the first two minutes, but I suppose that is the advantage of slavery—if you are in charge. All this work went into the preparation for the afterlife.

At the moment of death, the pharaohs believed that the soul would be liberated to the heavens, but only in part. A portion of the soul remained with the body, which was why the pyramids were built—to store the treasures and house the bodies of pharaohs after death. They believed in building for immortality, and they required all these resources for the afterlife.

The concepts of spirituality and an afterlife were not unique to the Egyptians and the Greeks. Many cultures have a story about an afterlife. We stand where we are today because of our spiritual foundation. Our concepts of good and evil and our moral codes are not based on physical or emotional principles, but rather on eternal, spiritual principles. With these, we transcend our basic animalistic instincts.

These truths may be culturally based. Our spiritual views will be mostly influenced by our cultural background. When it comes to the afterlife, there are many beliefs and, as much as they are varied and differ, they are unanimous in accepting that we do not end when this life is done.

Much of our modern idea of spirituality is based on the teachings of the major historical religions. The Hindu and Buddhist faiths believe in an afterlife where the spirits are reincarnated until they achieve perfection and escape from this earthly lower cycle of death and destruction. There you either become as one with Brahma if you are a Hindu or enter Nirvana as a Buddhist. The Islamic, Jewish and Christian faiths believe in an afterlife where you will face judgment and be accountable to a single, omnipotent God. The notion of spirituality is not lost on 85% of the world's population who have a religion.

Even for the non-religious or spiritually disinterested, spirituality still shapes our language and contemporary lifestyles. We may refer to demons, but what else are they other than eternal evil spiritual entities? Equally, angels are enlightened spiritual beings. What about the countless supernatural phenomena that people will happily accept as real—like bad luck from breaking a mirror, your star sign influencing your life, or how some people believe in ghosts? How do people explain astral projection, divination, prophecy, cursing, magic, witchcraft, levitation, Ouija boards, or other practised spiritual experiences?

The main argument against spirituality is that it has not been proven: "Show me God and then I will believe!" This demand for evidence fails because it assumes that the spiritual world operates like the physical one. The spiritual dimension is not temporal or limited by the laws of physics, and it cannot be explained by science. Science often incorrectly refutes the reality of the spiritual world, but before we unconditionally accept this 'lack of evidence', we need to understand how the scientific process actually works.

Science uses a process called 'the scientific method' to verify a fact. This requires collecting relevant data to prove or refute a hypothesis about a specific question. It starts by asking a question:

- Is the sun hot?
- Is hydrogen explosive?
- Do people feel fear as they are dying?

Those three questions all deal with things that can be measured. The data that are collected can help us answer the question. We can measure the indirect temperature of the sun and draw a conclusion that the sun is hot. It is possible to ignite some hydrogen, but the careless scientist may not be around to confirm the experiment after the explosion. We can ask questions in qualitative research to confirm that people are afraid of dying.

But when it comes to spirituality, we have no way of measuring data. In 1907, Duncan MacDougal set out to weigh the mass of the soul by measuring the change in weight when people died. He concluded that after death had occurred, the body had lost 21.3 grams of its mass and hence this is the weight of the soul. His research was flawed according to the scientific method, because there was nothing physical he could measure or point to and say, "this is a soul" and show *it* was the mass that had changed. This research was probably more important for proving evidence that spirituality is not measurable, yet.

If you cannot collect or measure data, it is bad science to say, "There was nothing to measure, so that means there is nothing." It would be accurate to say, "Without data we cannot draw any conclusions." It would also be a different story if there were data to prove that spirituality did not exist, but there isn't.

When it comes to spirituality, we cannot rely on scientific evidence and we need to look elsewhere. We have touched on spirituality in culture, folklore and religion. While these can help, they do not provide us with contemporary evidence of spirituality.

Is there any evidence that we are spiritual beings, and that we exist in an afterlife? Yes! There is evidence that supports the idea that at the time of death, our spirit leaves our physical body and returns to God. We do not die but merely change dimensions, trading this physical dimension for a spiritual dimension.

We need to ask those who know.

Chapter 18

Near-Death Experiences (NDEs)

George Foreman, the former heavyweight boxing champion of the world, had just lost a fight. But he'd lost on purpose; the match was rigged. In the changeroom after the loss, George was chatting to his team when suddenly he dropped down dead. His spirit left his body and he descended into hell or a place of terrible torment.

He called out to God and recalls being pulled up out of hell by this huge hand of God. He had died as a mean, non-believing man and returned to life as a new man, a man of faith. In his book, *God in my corner: A spiritual memoir*, he describes this remarkable event before going on to describe its consequences and his changed life after the event. His encounter with spirituality transformed his life. Against all odds, he went on to once again become the heavyweight boxing champion of the world.

In 1999 in a separate NDE, Dr Mary Neale, an orthopaedic surgeon, set off along with her husband and some friends on a white-water kayaking expedition to a remote part of Chile. While on a Grade Five rapid, a team member with little kayaking experience forced Mary off course.

She went over the rapid and plunged into a deep pool below with tons of water gushing over her. Submerged and trapped underwater by the sheer force of the water pouring on top of her, Mary couldn't move or free herself and drowned. As Mary died, she felt her spirit leave her body. In her book she elaborates on this experience, describing her consciousness and awareness of the events unfolding around her, as well as the spiritual experience she has with other human spirits and with God.

Dr. Eben Alexander was a neurosurgeon known as the 'master' of scepticism about spirituality and life after death, and he experienced his own NDE. In his 2012 book, *Proof of Heaven: A neurosurgeon's journey into the Afterlife*, he describes his experience as being undoubtably in a spiritual dimension. He goes on to describe our spiritual ignorance and compares our spiritual understanding to that of a chimpanzee trying to comprehend calculus.

There are many, many stories of people who have died and live to tell the tale. These accounts have been refuted by scientists and explained as the last fizzing of the dying brain. But dying brains do not work. The higher functioning reported by those who have had an NDE argues that there is an additional source of consciousness: our soul.

NDEs may vary in minor details from person to person, and personality to personality, but in essence they all share the following characteristics.

A life-threatening illness or injury causing death
You can't die of nothing; something has to end this life. Those who have had an NDE have all experienced some catastrophic medical event, and the associated suffering that goes with it. At the time of death, the point at which the spirit leaves the body, all the pain and suffering associated with the event stops.

A sense of being dead
People who have had an NDE are aware that they have died. They are left in no uncertainty about this.

An out-of-body experience
Those who have had an NDE describe the spirit or soul leaving the body. They sometimes hang around for a while, and witness their lifeless body, and the efforts to resuscitate them. They possess consciousness and awareness even though they are not in their body. Independently of the body, the soul is conscious; it is aware.

A journey
Once the soul has departed the body, it undertakes a fantastical journey to another dimension. This is often described as being through a tunnel of white light.

Sometimes, the events of their life are played out before them, replaying the past and showing all the details of the things they have done—good and bad. Some are accompanied by friends and family members who have died, others describe angels.

A destination
Those who have died either arrive at a place of such great joy and beauty, and so filled with peace and love that they are overwhelmed with a magnitude of these feelings unimaginable on Earth. There is no pain or suffering here, only bliss. This is Heaven, and those who arrive here have no desire to be back on Earth. There is no comparison between the place they find themselves in, and the place they have left behind. Everyone wishes to stay.

However, some report a very different experience, finding themselves arriving at a destination that can only be described as Hell. This is a place of terrible suffering, full of darkness and demons, and with an atmosphere of torment and fear. It appears in the description of many NDEs.

A return
Those who have had an NDE are instructed by a greater spiritual authority to return to their physical bodies. There is no thought of not doing this, or thoughts of rebellion. They return, often with a mission to complete a specific task. This is a reluctant journey back for those who had gone to what could be described as Heaven. They often

report a release from the pain associated with their injuries as their spirit left the body, and now the pain's return as the spirit re-enters their lifeless body.

A period of adjustment

The effects of an NDE are profound, and many struggle to readjust to the gloominess and dullness of everyday life on Earth. After experiencing the exquisite joy of Heaven, nothing here seems to spark excitement or joy for them any longer. Often those who have had an NDE experience a spiritual transformation, aflame with the knowledge that they have a future and that this future is in Heaven with God.

No more fear of death

For those who during an NDE encountered the measureless love of God and know that death is no more than a homecoming, there is no more fear of death. It is not the great unknown any longer. Life here is a period of separation from the greater life and joy that awaits us after this one. In that, there is hope.

NDEs offer compelling evidence that there is a part of us that continues to exist after the physical body has died. They are first-hand accounts of this spiritual dimension. Would the testimony of an NDE survivor stand up in a court of law? Is their testimony reliable? We would scoff if it was the only story. But if NDEs are reproducible, with so many people saying similar things, it becomes more difficult to dismiss this evidence as nonsense.

The question is, do we believe this nonsense? Is this evidence of spirituality compelling enough for us to consider the new elephant in the room: our spirituality?

If so, the issue is no longer that we die, but rather that we will continue to live on in some form after this body has expired. This might be an unwanted intrusion into our hope for a blissful end to everything, one where all the lights go out and then it is 'all over red rover'. But if it is not over when we die, if it is only beginning, then we have a spiritual responsibility to know what to expect, and what to do, when we cross over into the next life.

Chapter 19

Spiritual Awakening

For me, the essence of spirituality is the recognition that we are spiritual beings with souls.[2] On the one hand, this definition simplifies matters because it avoids the contention around religion. On the other hand, it complicates matters because, if we are spiritual beings that possess souls, we have a responsibility to take care of our spirits.

What do you know about your spirit? It is not as if we have lessons at school on the anatomy of our spirits and how to look after them. What does it look like? What does it do? What does it need? How do you take care of this thing that suddenly belongs to you and is essentially you? When did you last glance in the spiritual mirror to see how you are doing?

In simplest terms, your spirit is your eternal breath and the vital essence within you. We each have a spirit, and it has the following characteristics.

---

2   Throughout, 'soul' and 'spirit' will be used interchangeably to reflect the eternal and spiritual component of our being, although technically they are separate terms.

It is our essential being

Our spirits are part of us and make us who we are. Spirit determines our nature and character. It can be described as the heart or psyche of a person. It is probably located in our belly or chest rather than in the head. It is where we feel yearning and strong emotion. When we are heartbroken, or when we are ecstatic, we feel it in our souls or spirits. When we encounter God, it is our soul that meets with Him.

Our spirits may be dormant and need to wake up

There is a requirement to have a spiritual awakening before spiritual things become relevant. Mostly, because our spiritual components are not visible, we are unaware that they even exist or have a role and a function. The Christian concept of being born of the spirit or 'born again', reflects the need for this awakening to happen before we can be spiritually aware.

Our spirits are invisible

Don't try to find your spirit, you won't be able to. It is invisible, and like the air it has no substance to it. We have never seen our souls, just like we have never seen the wind. But we can feel the presence of the wind and understand its nature by the effect it has on things, and we can do the same with our souls.

Our spirits are immortal and eternal
Our spirit does not die, it endures. At the time of death, the living spirit leaves the lifeless body as it moves on into the next dimension.

The spirit is priceless
Because the spirit endures forever, it is priceless. If your spirit is only worth a miserable penny a day, it does not take long to realise that, over the course of eternity, the value of your spirit is priceless. You have been given a high value, and your value lasts forever.

The spirit has consciousness
Those who have had an NDE describe their consciousness continuing to exist after their death. They are aware of things happening around them; they experience sensation and feeling and retain the memories of the events they have experienced after they return to their physical bodies.

The spirit has an identity
Following death, souls maintain their identity. In the stories about NDEs, those who have died describe being recognised by people as the person they knew in life despite nothing of their physical body being present. We will recognise those we know in the afterlife, and they will recognise us. We already have a spiritual identity.

The nature of the spirit is forged by life and choice

As humans, we have the unique gift of choice. In life, our choices determine who or what we are. We get to say yes or no to the choices life offers us. Those without choice are slaves. We sometimes get to choose our friends, our partners, our homes and our occupations. We also get to choose the morals that we use to guide us in issues that affect our spirit. We get to choose between right or wrong. We get to choose what God we will have faith in. The nature of our choices affects the nature of our spirits.

Our spirit is accountable

Almost all religions agree on the following three points:

- at the time of death, the spirit leaves the body
- there is a form of judgment and accountability for the way the spirit conducted itself in this life
- based on this, there is either a reward or punishment awaiting the spirit after death.

The spirit is not independent, we are not alone

If the spirit is accountable in death, the next question must be: to whom? Who gets to judge us and the way we have lived our life? By implication we are subject to authority at the time of death.

We may have been in control of our affairs on Earth, but we may not be in control of our affairs after Earth.

The spiritual experience

From a natural perspective, we are 'seriously disabled' spiritually. We cannot see, smell, feel or hear anything in the spiritual dimension. While the spiritual world may be all around us, all the time, we are mostly blissfully unaware of what is going on around us spiritually. We need help.

We may have had some spiritual experiences without being aware of it.

Those who explore their spirituality and choose to open their eyes to the spiritual realm may be astounded to discover the depth and breadth of beliefs and practices out there. In South Africa, witch doctors can curse a person and evil spirits will do their bidding to bring about harm and even death. Those who practise sorcery or witchcraft or perform divination are aware of the realm of spiritual entities that do their bidding. Those who have religious faith are aware of the inexplicable spiritual events that occur because of their belief.

The spirit ultimately meets with God

Whether you believe in one of the monotheistic gods of the Christian, Jewish or Islamic faiths, worship the great Brahma of the Hindu faith or achieve the state of Nirvana through the teachings of Buddha, at the moment of death you encounter something greater than yourself. Whatever form it takes, you will get to say hello to your God.

Spiritual responsibility

With all this to consider, it is not unusual to feel a sense of disquiet about the nature of this invisible realm and your status in it. Is it well with your soul? Do you have an expectation of reward in the afterlife, or are you perhaps feeling a sense of dread about the possibility of not dying totally?

This may be a very important moment; the realisation that, as spiritual beings, our innermost nature is exposed, and this exposure is to God. As spiritual beings we have a responsibility for the welfare of our spirits. Is there something we can do to make up for lost time, poor choices and spiritual blunders? Of course, there is!

Chapter 20

Exposure To God

This is such an impossible chapter to write because anyone who puts forward an opinion about God is bound to get something wrong. I don't only mean from a religious perspective, but rather that we are incapable of fully understanding or knowing God.

Over time, our attempts to understand a greater being have come up with so many gods and so many possibilities. On the one hand, God may be shaped by our perceptions. On the other hand, God is, by nature of being God, independent of our opinions.

With more than 2500 religions and counting, I am sure I may have missed a few possibilities along the way, so please bear with me. I also respectfully apologise if I am treading on any toes by discussing God. We cannot be mature in considering death if we do not consider God.

Whether we are religious or not, we probably all have a concept of God. And we will know this god by what we choose to worship. Worship is such a weird word. It means 'to show reverence or adoration', and although it is implied that this is in the context of a deity, it doesn't need to be.

It is easy to identify who you've made *your* God by looking at what the purpose of your life has been. What has driven you? What do you pay attention to and give homage to above everything else? What do you love more than anything else? What can't you live without? What are you prepared to die for?

I have my own faith, and nothing would give me more pleasure than to share it with you, but there is a time and place for everything. If you want to know what I think and believe about God, you will have to read through to the epilogue. For now, please bear with me, tongue in cheek, as we consider possibilities of God.

The belief that there is no God or any need for a God

Some believe God is not relevant or required. They believe that they are self-sufficient in what they do. In the broadest sense, they are a god unto themselves, and their purpose and direction in life has been self-directed. As masters of their own destiny, they are only guided by concrete facts, science, information, and knowledge. They see us only as biological entities, and as such, we are born, live and die. That's it, there is nothing more to consider. Spirituality is not real.

We all have our idols

Some of the gods we serve are created by us. We may not necessarily bow down and worship them in a religious sense, but our lives are dedicated to their service. There are many of these gods, and they shape us and make us who we are. There is the god of money and wealth. Those who serve this god have dedicated their entire lives to being rich and gaining possessions. They are identified by their wealth. For others, it is power that drives their actions and behaviour. They need to be in charge, regardless of the cost. Others devote their lives to being famous and loved. Still others devote their lives to their professions or skills.

Whatever we make our idols, these things define us. While we wouldn't ever call them our gods, they demand our attention and direct our lives, and they are something worth dying for.

The force

"May the force be with you." Some believe God is not a person or a distinct entity, but is an energy, a light, a source of goodness, brilliance and enlightenment. We seek to take on the nature and character of this god by living in harmony with the life force of the universe, surrendering our own wants and needs and letting go of our identities, until we eventually become one with the light. This force is ever-present, and it gives life and light to us all. It is a part of everything and what connects everything.

The force is non-discriminatory, judges no one and accepts all. The beginner is as welcome as the master, for we are all ultimately on the same journey, even if some of us take longer to get there.

The multitude of gods

You need to bring your Rolodex along to keep track of these gods. They are both major gods and demigods, good and evil spiritual forces, the demonic and angelic—all out to influence your life. As you pass from one life to the next, and the next, they add spice—some helping you up to greater enlightenment, and others pulling you down.

If you worship the right god enough, you will get ahead, become a saintly person and, as with the force, eventually become enlightened. But if you neglect your duties to your god, you will regret it. The advantage of having so many gods is that you can never run out of gods.

The malevolent gods

These gods are scary. They demand worship and absolute obedience. Their anger is a terrible thing and with it comes punishment. If you do not pay homage and give your service to these gods, misfortune will befall you. The crops will fail. You will be struck down with plague, disease and disaster. You better watch out; few can be worthy, and you are at risk of failing every day. If you ever do make it to paradise, it will be by the skin of your teeth. Most other people won't make it, and they don't deserve to, either. Those who do not obey will be punished.

The benevolent gods

These gods are good. These gods are only love. They are there to serve us. These gods have our best interest at heart above everything else. With them there is no risk of punishment or accountability because everything will be just fine. It is easy to worship them because they are always good, giving and kind. You can never go wrong because these gods are on your side. These gods may go as far as sharing their divinity with you so that you may become like them, a true son or daughter of god.

All you have to do is present yourself and these gods will come running to serve you.

The moment of truth

While it may be fun to make fun of God, God is no laughing matter. If we have a destiny to meet with God, we need to know and be confident about what we believe about God.

The following are the things I believe about God:

- God is holy—there is no impurity with God.
- God is the creator—everything that exists originated with God.
- God is sovereign—He has the final say in all things.
- God is love—but this love comes with consequence and accountability.
- God is undefinable: beyond our comprehension or imagination.
- God is the source of all life.
- God is interested in you because He made you —you do belong to Him.

- God is waiting for you to meet with Him —the sooner the better—that's how we build relationships.

What are the statements you can confidently make about your God? I know many of my friends would not agree with all of these statements, and that is fine. Our understanding of God is not something we can know to be true, but something we can only believe to be true. Faith is at the heart of believing. And, when it comes to our faith and our belief system, the most critical question is, "Do you trust your God?"

Trust and faith are different. As a child I could not swim, and I was afraid of the 'big' pool. My father would stand in the scariest deep end of the pool and say to me, "Jump! I will catch you."

At the time, having faith in my father meant believing my father would try to catch me, but it was only by jumping that I demonstrated that I trusted he would do so. Trust requires a relationship and knowledge about the character of the person you are committing yourself to. It was easy to trust my dad, I knew him, and as much as I was afraid, I was able let go of my secure position and launch myself into his safe hands.

I think this is what Mrs. Blades had when she faced death. She had a life surrendered to a God that she knew. She not only believed in her God, but she also trusted Him. When it came to leaping from this life into the next, she knew she was in safe hands. She not only knew *what* she believed in; she knew *who* she believed in.

When it comes to the welfare of your soul, are you in safe hands? If you feel insecure, or have more questions after finishing this book, you can get in touch with me at admin@dyingtounderstand.com.

Chapter 21

Into The Storm

There is a huge difference between being a spectator and a competitor. As a lounge chair professional, I can tell you exactly what's going wrong with the game and how to improve it and win. Making my New Year's resolution to get fit and lose weight was easy; I didn't even break into a sweat. Deciding to run a marathon is an easy task if you only ever think about doing it.

One of our mind's best tricks is to con us about having done something when we haven't actually done anything at all. We get all the benefits; we feel pumped up. We are ready for anything the moment we put on our running shoes—all kitted out for a 10 km jog and good to go. We're a very different and sorry sight when we return home hours later.

The same con job occurs when we think about dying. On the face of it, it might seem quite easy, but there are several things we must contend with along the way. By now we may have summoned the courage to face death, accept our fate as mortals, have a good story ready to go, and understand the physical, emotional and spiritual challenges of dying. We may feel we are ready, but all this has just been the warmup, the pep talk, the pre-game stretches. The reality is that dying is going to be difficult.

In the process of dying, the physical body is going to break down. It will malfunction according to the nature of the disease. This will all be something new, unexpected, unpredictable, inconvenient, frustrating, depressing and just plain awful. So, we need a strategy of some sort. Emotions will run high and low—they will even be explosive at times. Exhaustion will set in, and sometimes, everyone will be on edge. There are spiritual issues to contend with, and for many, these are profound tests of faith. Why has God abandoned me? Why does God not hear me? Where is God when I need Him?

We may now know the theory about dying, but the reality is not easy. It is messy. Dying is hard work. It can be a very long and bumpy journey for all involved and because of that we need some kind of game plan or strategy. Why bother, you may wonder? Why go to all that effort and fuss if it's all just going to turn out the same in the end?

We need to make an effort because dying affects more than just one person. Many people feel its impact: partners, wives, husbands, children, friends, family, colleagues, mothers, fathers and even the gardener. There is an opportunity to get it right for everyone's sake.

We all have different circumstances, and it is not possible to have a one-size-fits-all scenario, but here are some starting points to help define a strategy.

You are going to feel unwell, more and more

Expect to feel unwell. If it never happens, consider it a bonus.

Earlier we spoke about disappointment and how it is linked to expectation. It is here where we need to lower our expectations. We can't expect our body to be awesome anymore. In dying, our body is going to let us down; don't let this come as a surprise. With cancer, common symptoms are fatigue and pain, as well as any side effects of treatment. Be ready for all these in the same way you would be ready for stormy weather—pack an umbrella.

As health deteriorates, more and more time is spent at the doctors, in hospitals and in clinics. Make space for this in your daily preparation. Anticipate which days of the week are going to be doctor days. Work around your medical appointments to plan time for yourself and schedule 'me time'.

Don't be stupid when it comes to pain

Pain is a common symptom in advanced illness, but it serves no purpose. This pain doesn't tell you anything you don't already know, so you don't need to put up with it.

One of the worst comments I hear is, "I can put up with the pain." And my immediate comment is, "Why?" There are no medals for suffering pain. Pain is cruel. It takes away hope. It causes depression, limits function, decreases immunity and limits our participation in life. Pain hurts—if you hadn't already noticed.

Taking drugs to manage the pain is a good thing. Some people can get addicted to the drugs they need for pain, but it is uncommon and if it is terminal pain, does an addiction really matter in comparison to alleviating suffering? Opioids such as morphine are *good* drugs to take if you have pain. They may cause side effects, such as constipation and nausea, but we can anticipate these and manage them with appropriate medication.

If the drugs make you feel unwell, manage the symptoms, change the drugs, find alternative pain treatments, but please, please, please, never put up with pain. Always seek to be as pain-free as possible. Sometimes it is not possible to be totally pain-free, and sometimes, we have to accept some pain. But a 4 out of 10 on the pain scale is better than a 6. Aim low when it comes to pain.

Run your own race - tell others to back off

One of my friends had advanced breast cancer and didn't want her husband to be prescribed morphine when he was diagnosed with painful and advanced lung cancer. This was because *she* did not need to take morphine for her cancer symptoms. She did not experience pain, so obviously, she (incorrectly) concluded that he should also not have pain.

Our personal experiences and opinions do not count if we are not the patient. Just because something is right or wrong for us doesn't mean it is the same for someone else. No one can tell someone else how they should be feeling. It is only the patient who knows how they are feeling.

Well-meaning loved ones often do not understand the physical limitations of a failing body. It is impossible to get better by trying harder. Physical failure is the nature of illness, those who expect things to be like they were before need to back off.

With advanced cancer, we get to run our own race and do it our way.

Be content with small wins—give your body a break

We all have high expectations when it comes to our health because we have been so used to good health in the past. There is often enormous frustration about not being able to achieve what was previously so achievable. You might have been able to run a marathon, but now you can only walk 200 metres. You could eat a horse, but now you can only manage a few nuts and half a banana. Don't be resentful if your body cannot do what it has always done. A few nuts is a good effort, and perhaps a banana in a smoothie is the way to go. If you need a nap, take a nap. Give your body a break. It will be thankful.

Don't be a hero—admit when you are taking a beating

As the body malfunctions, it takes more time and more effort to manage. Symptoms may be debilitating. If they are, you are allowed to be debilitated. Don't be a hero and suffer unnecessarily. If your body is not able, it is not able. Be honest about how you feel.

If you can't mow the lawn, then don't. If you can't

go to work, then don't. If you can't do the dishes though, it is no excuse unless you check with your partner first. Jokes aside, speak to those around you about the changes in your body and about what you can and can't do. Negotiate a new work schedule with yourself and with the team.

Love yourself

As your body changes during illness, it may begin to look different. Weight loss is a common symptom of advanced illness, and this may seem ugly to you. Remember you are far more than your body. You are the person you have always been. Continue being that awesome person. Love who you are.

Make space

When you are feeling sick you do not always have great coping skills. Having to chitchat with friends when you are feeling nauseous or experiencing diarrhoea is not much fun. Feel free to tell your friends to 'buzz off' if you are not feeling well or limit visits to time slots that work for you. This is particularly important when everyone is coming to say their final goodbyes. Keep these visits short and meaningful, there is no need to relive the past 70 years in an afternoon.

Pace yourself

Dying is a marathon, not a sprint. As with all marathons, there are uphills and downhills, times to walk and rest, and times to jog a bit faster. It takes endurance and effort to run a marathon, and it is the same with dying. Only plan how you are going to get to the next base, complete the next 100 metres or get to the next refreshment stop—not how you are going to get through the whole race.

Illness comes in waves, there are good moments and bad moments, and they are often unpredictable. Have a strategy to roll with the punches and punch back when you can.

Know what to expect

Knowing what to expect when dying is useful. From a cancer perspective the final changes in the body are predictable. Discuss your symptoms with your doctor and ask questions. Make up a list of questions as they come to you. Being prepared for what may happen allows you to take a proactive role in minimising the symptoms when they do occur.

Get help

Don't do dying on your own. It is not a DIY project, so get help from the professionals.

One of the things that freaks people out the most is when they are referred to palliative care. If palliative care is available, make use of these amazing specialists who know a lot about dying and how to support the failing body.

People get mixed up between terminal care and palliative care. Palliative care is much broader, and it covers all the aspects of medical care when curative treatment is no longer an option. This also includes terminal care at the very end of the journey.

One of my patient's daughters was very angry and indignant when I suggested a referral to palliative care, as she thought it meant terminal care.

"How can you just sit there and say that? How can you be so cruel and unfeeling?"

I like to think of the palliative care team as the 'obstetric team' of dying. They should be there from the beginning of an incurable illness right through to the very end.

There are often many resources in the local community, find out about them and make use of them if you can and if you want to.

Understand the process

The process of dying takes time. This is longer for some than for others. With cancer, we can slow it down with treatments such as chemotherapy, immunotherapy or biological therapy. Good diet, exercise, prayer, meditation and alternative therapies may all also help. While these may slow down the process of dying, they can't prevent it forever.

As the body gets weaker there will be less opportunity to do the things that need to be done. Get in and do the hard work up front. We discuss all the things that need to be done, such as advanced directives and funeral planning later. Don't put these off too long or there will not be any fuel left in the tank to do them.

Know when it is time to let go

Angus had advanced cancer and came in to see me about receiving further radiation treatment. His body was broken from the cancer and the effects of treatment. He had a new cancer in his brain and was in the terminal phase of dying. I explained to him that his life was ending and that he was dying—it was time to let go. I talked to him about how, at the end of the journey, it was important to allow dying to happen. There is a time to accept, to unclasp the hand that holds onto life and to trust the next step. There is no shame in throwing in the towel. No one is victorious over death.

I tried to convince Angus that now was the time to be at peace, to spend the last days in the company of the ones he loved and to relax into the final phase of life. He refused my advice and demanded radiation treatment. Sadly, he died on the second day of treatment. His effort was not heroic, it was unnecessary. There will be a time when giving yourself permission to let go is an important step in permitting yourself to have a good death.

Giving up on life when it is time for death is not a failure, it is wisdom. Tell those you love it is okay for them to go. Bless them and give them space to let go and die. Often leaving the room for a while is all that is needed for those we love to leave for the next great adventure. Please give death permission to pass when it is time.

Be nice to the team

Few people die alone. Most are fortunate enough to have

friends and family caring for them on this journey. These carers also feel pain, suffer, get tired and need a break. Be nice to them.

Manage your feelings
Feelings come and go. Don't make rash decisions or say harsh words when your feelings are out of control. Take time out if you have to. Understand that those around you will also have strong feelings. If your emotions are destroying relationships, please ask for help.

Finish your story your own way
Remember to write your own narrative. Think about good ways to end this life for when this life has to end. Think about the incredible possibilities in the next life. Be deliberate about changing a negative narrative into a positive prediction. You don't have to write a bad ending for yourself.

Make peace and bury the hatchet
We all make mistakes in life. Sometimes these are terrible mistakes, and we carry the burden of them with us forever. When life is ending, find forgiveness and give forgiveness. As much as possible, make past wrongs right.

Explore your spirituality
Make every effort to be spiritual. Talk to spiritual people you trust. Take the time to take care of your soul and

spirit. Have a conversation with God or, if you don't like speaking, write God a letter—it may sound crazy, but for some people, writing it may be the key to unlocking a conversation with God.

Be a legend and leave a legacy

You can't take it with you when you die, so why not share it now while you can? Share your stories, tell people about your life, write a journal. Get in touch with us at admin@dyingtounderstand.com to tell us how you feel, share what bothers you and ask questions, so that we can all learn about this journey. Share your experiences with us. Please give us feedback.

Be flexible

Did I mention that things change a lot during the dying process? Be flexible. Any of your watertight and foolproof plans might need to be changed without warning. Sorry, that's in the nature of the journey. Be prepared to modify and change your plans.

Don't feel you need to stay loyal to a plan once you've committed. This is the time for having as many plans as you need. If you had decided not to have chemotherapy, but are having second thoughts, don't die a martyr—change your mind if you have to. If you decided you would never go into hospital care, but it becomes clear that you need to be there, please go. No one is keeping score, and if they are, my recommendation is to cheat.

Treat yourself

When all else has been considered, don't forget to treat yourself. Just because things are not going well sometimes, does not mean that they won't ever go well. Find those moments where the sun does shine and, even if it does not shine, find a way to sing in the rain. Even on a bad day, try to find those things that make you happy. Have some of that exquisite hand-crafted chocolate, go for a massage, just do what it takes to make your journey a little bit more fun. Don't skimp on being spoilt. Pamper yourself—after all, you are worth it.

We have covered a lot of ground by this point, and I hope that a plan is coming together. There are not only a lot of things we need to know; there are also a lot of things we need to *do*. We now turn to the practical aspect of dying.

Chapter 22

Action Stations

Dying involves a whole lot of 'things to do' that need to have been completed by the time death actually arrives. Some of them are good things, and some are very important. As with any approaching storm, the difference between a disaster and a passing inconvenience is the preparation.

Queensland is a beautiful part of Australia, but it does have the occasional cyclone that pays it a visit. The cyclones are never a surprise, everyone can see them coming for miles, and the Bureau of Meteorology gives timely warnings about the approaching storm. Houses are built to cyclone rating standards, so that they provide shelter.

Our last cyclone warning turned out to be a false alarm, but we would have been fully prepared to face the storm. Loose fittings and furniture were packed away. Trampolines, chairs, tables, dog kennels and other items that could become airborne, were secured. Like little ants, we scurried to and fro making sure that everything would be safe before the storm hit, and then it was, "Hold on tight, here she comes!" In the end, the storm didn't come, but we would have been ready in the event it had.

Dying is much the same: the storm is coming and there are important things we need to do before it arrives. Even if the storm does not arrive this time, it will arrive at some time. Being prepared early is much better than scrambling to set our affairs in order at the last minute.

The things we need to set in order are personal matters. They are unique and important to us. In life we gather information and store it to use as we need it. We all carry secrets and if we do not share them, we will take them to the grave. This may be acceptable if they need to remain secret, but if they need to be shared and are not, they will be lost forever. There is a lot of information being lost every day because people forget to mention something important before they die. It may be trivial, such as the name of the school principal in grade 1, but it is no joking matter if it is the combination to the family safe.

In the hurly-burly of dying, there are last things and little things we may forget, and the consequences can be devastating for those left behind. Big things, such as a will, funeral planning and estate planning, may have all been done, but there is more information that is required to keep things from becoming chaotic for our loved ones after we have died.

In Australia for example, there is a great emphasis on privacy. It is near impossible to do a transaction on behalf of someone else. I cannot change someone else's mobile phone plan or social benefits or banking transactions without their permission. The only way around this is if they have pre-authorised me to do this, or if I have a joint account with them.

When Bert died, his defacto partner Grace had no access to his bank accounts until the estate settled. Grace, had to ask her parents for money to support her because at the time of death, the bank account became 'frozen' and totally inaccessible. It did not matter how many millions of dollars may have been in the account, because she had no access to the money.

There are many things to consider before the final whistle blows. These require thinking and action, and because they are unique for all of us, our suggestions can never be exhaustive. Here are some of the little things that need to be recorded and taken care of before end of life.

Lists of important people

Even in a close relationship, it is easy to take things for granted. Names of important people are mentioned but never deliberately recorded, and in the aftermath of death, when things are hazy, foggy and confused, it is even more difficult to try to recall who is who in the zoo.

The following are essential people, who need to be recorded, along with the details of who they are, their role and contact details:

- lawyer
- accountant

- next of kin
- priest/rabbi/imam/other religious contact
- employer
- banker
- financial planner
- go-to person (such as daughter, wife, friend)
- executer of the will
- names of relatives and children
- funeral directors
- others, such as friends or club members, who will need to be notified when you die.

Copies of important documents

If you are like most people, your filing system will be in a state of entropy—files, books, pamphlets and 'bits and pieces'—all waiting to be organised once procrastination has left the building. If this is the case, it certainly will be a challenge for those left behind to try to find out where the important documents are hiding, if they ever existed in the first place.

To be kind, please consider creating a folder containing a copy of the following documents to make it easier for those trying to tidy things up after death has visited:

- wills and testaments
- enduring power of attorney
- advanced directives
- bank statements of all accounts so that they can be closed or managed

- shareholding statements of all share transactions so they won't be missed or forgotten
- utilities accounts for change of ownership/cancellation
- property titles
- telephone accounts
- vehicle ownership registration
- insurances including life, building, car, and home insurance
- gun licences, other licences
- memberships that need to be cancelled
- list of assets and liabilities so that nothing is missed along the way
- other important information to tidy up loose ends after death has visited.

Important information

These are the things we most frequently take for granted. Those things in our heads that we know and never expect anyone else would want to know. Write them down so that they are available in the event of an emergency:

- computer passwords and login details
- PINs to banking accounts, apps, or devices
- combination to the safe
- critical information, such as where the gold is buried
- your favourite apple pie or beef stew recipe, so that it is not lost forever

- other critical information relevant to your life
- schema of your family tree as far as you can remember.

Important task list

There may be things that are outside of your will that you want people to consider when you have died. It may be a wish or more defined instructions, such as:

- pay Bob the $100 you owe him
- get rid of the Land Rover that you have been restoring for 20 years—it should go to Sam
- return the wheelchair to Mary.

Whatever you think needs to be done, jot it down and make a list. The list may grow and seem to be superfluous but do it. The biggest challenge in doing the list is just doing it. Procrastination is my best friend, and as much as it promises that it can wait for tomorrow, this is not true when time is running out.

Start with these steps:

Find someone you trust. This is usually a spouse, but it may be a good friend, or even a lawyer if you don't have friends you can trust. Give them the authority to act on your behalf. You need to nominate someone as an enduring power of attorney, if you have not done so already. The person with enduring power of attorney will be able to represent your interests, if you are no longer able to do so.

Share your life. If you have a single account of any sorts (bank, post office, mobile phone, utilities, insurance), make it a joint account, or give the person you trust signing rights and authorisation to act on your behalf.

Tell all. Get out a secret notebook and write down the following important information: the passwords to important websites, the combination to the safe, where the gold is hidden and who to contact in the event of an emergency.

Does your partner know how to log in to your share trading account or to your government social security site? Is your safe so secure that it can never be opened, or found for that matter? Who is the lawyer, financial advisor and go-to person if you die?

Keep making lists. List your assets and liabilities. If you still owe Uncle Bob money that he lent you, please tell someone so that Uncle Bob won't hate you forever because you never paid him back. Your partner may not know about your secret stash of bitcoin—so write it down, so that it is not lost forever. It will be nice to know that nothing will get missed when it comes to the caring and sharing.

Be ready to cancel. Check your stuff. Things like banking statements are a world of information about where your money is disappearing on direct debits. Make sure that there is a way to turn them off after you no longer need the goods or services. The *Financial Times* won't care that you have died. They will keep delivering the news to you and charging a fee. Make sure these things end when you end.

Go over it again. Is there something you may have missed? If you live alone, your children may be keen to know where the car keys are kept, who the dog needs to go to, who gets to keep the family portrait, and how to switch off the lights—the last one out especially needs to know this. Think about it and make your list.

Don't hide your secret list. Once you have made the list, please keep it safe and share it with the person you trust. It will make the world a much happier place if you take the time to do this before you die. The list is not about you, it is about those you love and leave behind. If you care about them, start your list today.

Once you start, it is easy to keep going. But lists are not enough, and action items won't matter unless the important things that need to be done are done professionally.

Chapter 23

Communicating Legal & Financial Matters

One of the advantages of being alive is that you can communicate. You can tell others what you think. If you have ever played the game Pictionary, you will know how frustrating it is not to be able to communicate. Try to say something only using drawings, and it is fun seeing how wrong this can end up. Without proper communication, things can go wrong very quickly.

Communication is a skill we take for granted. At the top of the communication master-skill ladder are those who are so good at communicating that they think people can read their minds. This is usual in close personal relationships, such as marriages, where assumed communication occurs.

- Didn't you know I wanted a cup of tea?
- I didn't want you to plant the bush so close to the wall.

- I needed my shirt for the meeting tonight.
- I thought you knew we needed more cat food.

Once you get past the level of grand master and expert communicator, the rest of communication seems quite straightforward. It may seem easy to respond to a direct question, such as "Do you want Margaret to have the car after you die?" However, there are many minor details that need to be considered, such as which Margaret you were thinking of, and which car you had in mind.

How difficult can it be? Well, it turns out, very difficult. We often don't think about the importance of good communication, because we assume that we will always be able to communicate and explain what we meant. But this is not always the case; there are occasions where we are no longer able to communicate. Death is the most obvious, but there are others. Illnesses requiring ventilation, stroke and dementia will also affect our ability to communicate. When we cannot communicate, the quality of our existing instructions is all that the others have left to go on. If we do not communicate them, or if we communicate them badly, there will be chaos.

My father-in-law, who was a bank manager, had to sometimes witness signatures and changes to wills and testaments. On one occasion he was called in to witness an apparent change in a man's will. The man was unable to communicate verbally, and when he asked the man if he wanted to change his will, the man vehemently shook his head indicating a resounding, "No!" The family tried to convince my father-in-law that the man always shook his head when he meant yes. Needless to say, the will was not altered.

You can rest assured that, unless you clearly and painstakingly indicate your wishes, there will be a challenge. There are rogues and charlatans who will, by way of a good lawyer, try to 'un-communicate' what you thought you meant. In law, every full stop and comma has meaning.

We might say, "Let's eat Grandma", much to Grandma's distress, or "Let's eat, Grandma", to everyone's delight. In another example, when looking at the relative value of men and women, the meaning changes considerably between, "A woman, without her man is nothing," and, "A woman without her man is nothing."

It is not only about the punctuation. It is also important to know the law. In a family of three siblings, there were two sons who were close to their mother and cared for her. The third sibling, the daughter, was a drug addict who had left home and was no longer in contact with the family. The mother had no intention of leaving anything in her estate to her estranged daughter. When the mother passed away, being unfamiliar with the relevant laws and therefore not making provision for them, a third of her insurance policy was automatically passed on to the daughter. From a legal point of view there was nothing the sons could do about this, but if their mother had obtained financial and legal advice, this would have been prevented.

Knowing the legal 'ins' and 'outs' is important when it comes to communication. It is sometimes tempting to get a DIY will kit from the Post Office and do up your own will. This may be adequate if you have a very simple will and limited assets, but if things are complicated and you are expecting the vultures to gather after you have died, please get proper legal advice.

Good communication is required when you are in good health because bad health is never expected, but it may only be just around the corner. The following areas need attention so that you can have your say now, and that your wishes will be clearly followed at a time when you can no longer communicate.

Wills and testaments

When you die, what do you want to happen to all your possessions? If you don't have a will, someone you don't know and who is working for the court will get to decide, and every Tom, Dick and Harry will be able to make a claim on your goods. To protect your assets, and make sure they go to the people you love and intended to give them to, draw up a will and update it regularly. Close the door to the unwanted, like ex-wives, wayward children, fiendish siblings and, even sometimes, the good old government tax office. Make an appointment with a lawyer today.

Enduring power of attorney

Find someone you trust who can communicate and transact on your behalf if the situation arises where you haven't quite died but can no longer communicate. This is an essential task that you need to discuss with your lawyer; if you don't have a lawyer, find one.

If you have an enduring power of attorney, you have a fighting chance. Discuss with your lawyer about who this should be.

Advanced directives and 'not-for-resuscitation' instructions

What do you want the doctors to do with you if you are struck down with a permanent medical illness or catastrophe? In the sad case of Terri Schiavo, this ended up going badly and could all have been avoided if she had made her intentions clear about what should happen if she suffered a catastrophic medical event.

What do you want to happen if you suffered a non-life-ending stroke, but had no prospect of recovery?

I do not mind them having a go at keeping me alive if there is some hope, but if there is no change after 40 days, please disconnect me from life. Being connected to a device without any chance of a life is not for me. These are my instructions. What do you want?

One of the awkward conversations we have with patients who are admitted to the medical wards with an uncertain prognosis is the concept of a not-for-resuscitation or 'do not resuscitate' (NFR or DNR) order. If something goes wrong, do you want to be resuscitated?

There is a lot to this question, because resuscitation

probably involves the ICU, ventilation, medical bills and, possibly broken ribs if you have had CPR. And the original cause of the medical disaster may not even be fixable. This decision requires deep conversations with your doctor. By default, the medical team will do a full resuscitation, if you suddenly hit the wall. Is this what you want if there is no prospect of cure, and you'll get to do it all over again in a few weeks—even after a successful resuscitation?

Financial planning

You don't have to be a gazillionaire to need financial planning. Chances are you have worked hard all your life, and your assets and wealth are a reward for this hard work. The last thing you would want is to see some undeserving person take a huge bite out of your delicious estate.

This is why financial planning is so important. It is not only greedy people who want to make money when you die, the lovely government wants some too. Taxes and estate duties are a gentle way of ensuring you make a final contribution to the coffers of the government. Estate planning is a good way to legally divert the resources away from the government's coffers and towards those who are more deserving.

Then there are also issues of life insurance, key person insurance, trauma insurance, and I assume, where relevant, even pet insurance. These are considerations for the professionals and the aim is to provide a shield of protection for your loved ones in the event of loss. But, this usually needs to be in place before the loss occurs. It is never too soon to consider life insurance.

When it comes to all matters of communication, please take time to do them well. Make an effort to clearly communicate your will and desires in no uncertain terms before you need to and are no longer able to. There may be a need for very deep and difficult discussions.

Please get professional advice, but a word of caution first: not all professionals have your best interests at heart. Lawyers' fees can add up and be painful if you keep changing your mind about things. So, prepare in advance everything you want to discuss. Financial planners will sell you the world, with an insurance policy for every eventuality—including space travel if possible. Unless you plan on going to space, you don't need it. So, take along a stiff measure of scepticism and reality when you set off for advice.

The best bet is to go with someone you know and trust, or at least find someone who is recommended by a close friend or relative. If you have an ongoing relationship with a trusted advisor, such as an accountant, financial planner or lawyer, they are often able to coordinate and introduce you to the services you need. They can also refer you to helpful information about managing money, government systems and how the various industries work. Whatever your decision, don't neglect them or their advice. I have learnt from experience that money spent on good legal advice is always cheap compared to the money you will spend if you don't get legal advice.

Chapter 24

Funeral Planning

If funerals were not such sad affairs, they would be very entertaining. There is nothing quite like the chaos that occurs at a funeral. Typically, everyone is trying to do the right thing, but no one is sure what the right thing is. The best and worst of human emotions are on display, the heroes and villains arrive, and there may be drama. The set-up of intense emotions, intense people and no plot makes for potential comedy. To see it for what it is, you have to be able to step back and understand funerals.

The first thing to know is that something is going to go wrong. There will be a disaster, mishap or mayhem of some sort, and the sooner we realise this and relax, the easier it will be. There is no perfect funeral, unless you are royalty, and even then, I am sure things go terribly wrong that we are not aware of.

I remember the chaos leading up to my mum's funeral. We were all dressed up, tense, and ready to go to the church service, when there was a wild commotion outside. One of the neighbour's peacocks had inadvertently wandered along to the wrong side of the house—the wrong time and the wrong place—only to be savagely greeted by one of the guard dogs. It turned out badly for the peacock, for the neighbour, and for us as we, in the state of tense funeral anticipation, had to deal with a fowl tragedy. Although it was foul play for the peacock, it did help us to let off some steam. With this release of tension, the funeral went on quite well. We all survived, and life continued. That is the key thing to remember about a funeral—it is not the end of the world.

At a funeral, the worst that can happen has *already* happened. The person we love has already died. The tragedy is in the past. The funeral is not there to suffer that loss all over again.

There are three important considerations at a funeral, and if we focus on these, then funerals are not as impossible as they may seem.

The first purpose of a funeral is to dispose of the body, and for those with faith this is also a time to 'release' the soul so that it is unencumbered in the afterlife. These are important considerations, and each faith has its own set of rules and rituals when it comes to disposing of the body and farewelling the soul. It is important to take direction from religious leaders when it comes to the details of how to do this properly.

You're actual body is no longer required when you have died and if it is not disposed of, it causes a stink—literally. Generally accepted ways of disposing of the body are burial or cremation. Each has its own merits, costs and logistical considerations. For many, this is a personal choice, but often it is an uninformed choice. In the chaos of the death and funeral, the options are not always properly considered.

I, for example, would prefer a burial. I know they are more expensive, but I feel, as a citizen of the world, I am entitled to my own little patch of real estate. My reason for this is my experience of living in the United Kingdom for a year. Often, I would walk past an old church and churchyard and see the gravestones there and the inscriptions like *Joseph Watts, died in 1652*, or *Mary Spencer, died in 1885*. I saw these as an opportunity to think about the life they might have lived and what it had been like. For me, having a tombstone says, "I lived and my life mattered."

Cremations are quicker and easier, and there are fewer costs but once done and dusted, if you will excuse the pun, it is really all over. The advantage of a cremation is that it offers greater flexibility and freedom about the final resting place. People may have had a favourite place where they want their ashes to be scattered, or they may be in a foreign country and ashes are the easiest way to get home. Or for some it may simply be an unbearable thought to be buried underground. The final resting place is one of personal preference and choice but no one will know your wishes unless you tell them.

The second purpose of a funeral is to honour, celebrate and pay respect to the person who has died and the life they have lived. Our focus should be on honouring the dead, and not on being the centre of attention because we are attending the funeral of another person. Say nice things about the person who has died, and if you are planning your own funeral, be encouraged by the fact that people will say nice things about you.

The third important consideration is event planning. A funeral is a big event, and it will require all the event planning skills you can muster.

Some of the funerals I have been to have been a circus of overwhelming emotion because this was the expectation. Hold your horses—the purpose of a funeral is not to see the most emotionally distraught human beings on the planet. As much as I may want the whole world to mourn my death and expect that there may be weeks of darkness after my passing, I need to get a grip.

From a practical point of view, it is a day like every other day, there will be some challenges to get through, but at the end of it all the sun will still set and rise again the next day. It will not be the end of the world unless you want it to be.

For all of us, this will be our ultimate event, so why not make an effort to make it easy on those who will be there? Let's first consider the one thing you can easily do well.

Your funeral event planning

Before you can plan a funeral, it is important to set the scene. If you are generally liked, the people who love you are going to be sad at your funeral. If you are a horrible psychopathic person, there will be a general mood of happiness at your funeral. Work from the assumption that it will be a sad day and think about how you can make it easier for the people who are going to attend your funeral.

Remember you will not be there, so don't get all mushy and emotional about your funeral. It's not the funeral that causes your death; it's your death that causes the funeral. There is no reason to fear the funeral; it can do you no harm. Just do it—contact a funeral director if you are expecting a funeral and have a chat.

Your funeral will be a stock standard, boring event like every other funeral that the funeral directors do, unless you get involved. You need to be alive to get involved, so the sooner you do that, the better. Don't leave it until you are dead, like many others do.

A funeral is an event, so think about who will be there, the theme, catering, venue, accommodation for your guests and how to manage unwanted guests. Funeral directors are good at this, so make use of their expertise.

Why not have the final say at your funeral? Write your own eulogy and get someone to read it out on your behalf. Check it with your funeral director and family first. This, however, is not the time to confess sins or be unkind and have your final go at your ex-wife!

Remember that those who are at your funeral will feel sad, so try to think about ways to distract them from their sadness. Get rid of the clichéd funeral stuff. Get a coffin with designer patterns and play upbeat music, like 'We are the Champions' or 'When the Saints go marching in'. If you are a person of faith, make it known, celebrate the fact that you are in heaven, and all the suckers left on Earth have to wait for their turn. Plan a party, not a pity party.

Ask for help. Speak to your religious leaders about the expectations and requirements after death. Chat to the funeral directors if they are needed. Find someone who can help with event planning. Event planning is a big deal, so don't leave everything to the last minute. Time, or to be precise, the lack of time, is everyone's enemy when it comes to event planning. Do what you can now and have everything ready except the date of the event. Try to postpone that for as long as you want.

I know this is not easy. I know that even going to a funeral home violates all our principles of living and hoping to avoid death. I know that it shouts 'defeat' and that everyone who goes there feels like a bit of a loser. I know that funeral homes are often worse than we expected. I once went along to a funeral home to get advice about funerals and how it all works, and I must admit it was a traumatic experience. Based on that experience, I realise there needs to be a change in the game plan if you want to plan your funeral. It is why we need to have an 'up yours' attitude to funerals because, while we all need to have one, it should be on our terms.

The solution for me was to think of the funeral as a far and distant event. If you were planning your funeral for next year, or in five years' time, what would you want it to look like? Jot down some ideas. Be creative.

I know that within our cultures, this view may be insensitive, and I apologise for my cold-hearted approach to funerals. I do not mean to trivialise the loss, grief and sadness we feel when someone has died. These are all normal and to be expected, but they are not the only things that matter. If we keep believing and promoting the terribleness of death, it will always be a most terrible and fearful thing for us. If we are prepared to accept that death is normal, and our destiny, then we may as well make the most of it. After all, we only get to do our funeral once, so we may as well give it the best go we can.

The truth is that the issue around funerals is not the funeral in itself; it is that we have arrived at the part of life we have been avoiding all along. The terrible loss of death is in bereavement, and we will come to that, but first there is more work to be done.

Chapter 25

Make Provision For Illness And Death

Sorry, there are no free meals. Everything has a cost, and death and dying are no exception. It is unfair to not only have to suffer the indignation of dying, but to have to pay for it as well. It is not right, but that does not make it go away. So, we have to talk about money. You do not want to be left short-changed, after all is said and done.

In many countries, the government takes care of their own. They provide their taxpayers with good medical care, and there are no huge costs when it comes to this care. But they do not provide all the financial support that can possibly be required, and there are many additional costs to factor in when it comes to dying.

There are three important things to consider when it comes to money matters and dying. These are: decreased earnings, increased costs and bills, and the final costs relating to the estate and funerals.

Decreased earnings

As much as we may complain about having to go to work, we soon realise that there is a lot more to complain about if there is no work. With illness comes decreased earnings. Sick leave only goes so far, and there comes a point if you are unwell, that you will get laid off or made medically redundant. When the finance tap is turned off, the reserve tank can run dry very quickly. This financial stress can sometimes be worse than the stress associated with the illness itself. It is not easy to deal with being financially crippled by illness.

Would you be able to manage if your income decreased by half, or by the whole amount? Dealing with this will be impossible when it happens and making provisions for a rainy day is an important task. Talk to a financial planner today.

Increased costs

If you have a flourishing money tree growing in your garden this may not be such an issue, but if your money tree is weak and withering, this is a bumpy ride. When it comes to illness, there are the obvious costs of medical procedures, appointments, such as consultations and medication. Then there are the extras, like regular blood tests and imaging (MRIs, CT scans, PET scans, etc). As if that is not enough, doctors can seem to be a bunch of gangsters, referring you from one colleague to another, and each one charging like a wounded bull. They may add in dieticians or physiotherapy, and, as much as they provide an essential and important service, each time you go through the turnstile, it pings your credit card.

If you are armed with a strong medical insurance or are eligible to access a well-run government medical system, this may not be such a problem at first, but costs can add up. A co-payment here and there, an unexpected hospital admission or two, and there won't be any money left for cigarettes.

But these are not the only costs to consider. There are the hidden costs—the costs in fuel, parking and time. Because you are time-poor, and may not be physically capable, you may need a carer, cleaner or someone to mow the lawn. If you lose your licence due to illness, then it is taxi or Uber time. The list goes on. I know people who feel so frustrated by having to pay, and pay, and pay, that they take short cuts and avoid doctors' appointments if they are feeling well enough.

If you understand the system, there are better ways of getting things done. Do not despair just yet.

The cost of a funeral

You would think with all the grief and loss that occurs when someone dies, the funeral directors would be understanding and offer their service for free. It feels like it should be that way. Can't someone give us a break?

Sadly, they also have to make a living, and funeral directors charge a handsome fee to get rid of the body.

There are all sorts of hidden costs. A basic casket starts at *x* dollars, but then, if you want handles on it, that will cost another $100, and then the trimming to make it look fancier adds yet another $250, and on it goes. Flowers cost extra, and by the time you get the best possible (why wouldn't you want the best for the person you love?) the dollars are flying out the door. Burials are more expensive than cremations, so that's another cost to consider. When it comes to funerals, you need to apply a big foot to the brake and minimise losses.

The final costs

Depending on which country you live in, you may be subject to estate duties. For the privilege of dying, you will get to pay tax one more time. Add to this all the final fees and the medical bills that keep coming in after death, and it soon accumulates. It ends up being a fair-sized pile of money.

And as this is *your* money, here are some hints for making the most of the resources available and minimising the pain:

Financial survival tips

You are going to lose money when you die. Accept this, it is a fact of life. I know it is unfair, but I don't make the rules. If you want to win, you need to know the rules of the game.

Prepare for the rainy day

Seek advice from a financial planner and work out a way around the costs. Save up a little at a time so that if there are crazy costs, you have them sorted. It's like that extra stash of money you have when you are playing Monopoly. Land on Mayfair, pay and keep playing. Financial advisors may be able to give you hints about how to get ahead. If you are healthy, stay with your medical insurance if you can; don't cancel, even if it looks like a good idea.

Be stingy

Don't let costs blow out. Shop around for cheap deals. Ask if you can cancel unnecessary duplicate medical appointments. There is no need to see three of the same doctors in a week. Pick one doctor and go there. If you travel, try to tidy up all the business you have to do in that area at the same time. When it comes to funerals, go for the budget options. Don't be 'upsold' to have the best of the best. Talk them down to the cheapest and nastiest if you can. Don't fall for the sales pitch that only the best is good enough for you. Why not leave your best for your kids or to a cause you support, rather than the funeral director's bank account?

Get help

If you look around, there are probably going to be

many community groups that can help out with food parcels, lifts, care, and the list goes on. Seek advice from a social worker or your local religious or community organisations. They are there to help. Wisdom is asking for help when you need it. Being quiet is not going to solve any problems.

Make as much noise as possible

This is not a time to suffer in silence. Let all those who need to, know that you are suffering and let them know that it is terrible. The more you shout, the more you will get noticed, and it is human nature to pay attention to the loudest noise. It's sad, but true—the squeaky wheel gets the grease.

> I hate to be a kicker,
> I always long for peace,
> But the wheel that squeaks the loudest,
> Is the one that gets the grease.
>
> Josh Billings

Get some payback

If you have people who love you and care about you, why not consider a crowd-funding option? Often it is embarrassing to ask for help, and we are often too proud to admit that we are doing it tough financially. We don't want to be a burden to our families and friends, but they may be relieved and keen to help out once off as a group. Consider a proper crowd-funding campaign, rather than some half-baked fundraising venture.

Don't give up

It often seems like a good plan to sell off all your goods to fund the cost of illness. But, if you are compelled to downsize, do it on your terms and not as a fire sale. Be diligent in downsizing or moving into care by doing it earlier rather than later. Take the initiative when you realise that the season in your life has changed.

Some people really do it tough when their life is ending, so, if you can help in any way, why not become involved in your local community? It is amazing what can be achieved if we all do a little bit. If you can help, why don't you? And if you need help, why not ask?

Chapter 26

Palliative Care Heroes

I love the theme song in the movie *Ghostbusters*. I am sure most people will recognise it for its catchy tune and invitation to get the right people for the job, when the job is all about ghosts.

In the same way, the following words may be relevant when it comes to dying.

> When your body is malfunctioning and nothing seems to work,
> When your life is ending and before you have to croak,
> Who you gonna call?

The correct answer is the palliative care team. They are the health professionals you need when you are on the final lap of life. They are the superheroes who make dying easier. Just like the midwives and obstetricians support and care for the mum in the time of travail and birth, these fantastic people support and care for the dying body through the travail at the time of death. The sooner you meet with the palliative care team, the better the outcomes are expected to be.

Sadly, most people freak out when you mention palliative care or suggest a palliative care referral because of misrepresentations around death. There is also a great deal of misunderstanding over the terms: 'palliative care' and 'terminal care'.

Palliative care

Palliative care is a specialised field of medicine concerned with the care and welfare of the body, mind, and spirit at the end of life. These health professionals are neither uncomfortable with nor afraid of death. They see it as a final part of life. Their mission can be summarised in the statement from Edward Livingston Trudeau: "To cure sometimes, to relieve often, to comfort always."

Palliative care is about relieving and comforting when a cure is no longer available. As clinicians, we all ultimately fail in our promise to cure. We know that, and when that happens, we know that it is our obligation to care. Terminal care is that part of palliative care provided in the last days or hours of life, when death is imminent.

The discipline of palliative care is relatively new. It came from observations of the poor care people received at the end of life. It was obvious that more needed to be done for people in the terminal phase of life, and the aim of palliative care was to relieve suffering and distress. Dame

Cicely Saunders pioneered her ideas about a hospice in the 1950s and advocated for the relief of 'total pain' of the dying person in the context of family and a team approach.

In the 1960s, Elisabeth Kübler-Ross published *On Death and Dying*, and in doing so, kicked down the door of silence about death with her open and honest communication about dying. It was now possible to have a conversation about the meaning of death.

Today, palliative care is a recognised subspeciality of medicine, but very few people have access to a palliative care specialist. According to the World Health Organization (WHO), only 14% of people needing palliative care worldwide get it. If you have a palliative care service, you are in luck. Thankfully, most doctors are competent and confident in providing palliative care to cover most gaps.

Palliative care is the ultimate team effort. It requires doctors, nurses, social workers, bereavement counsellors, community workers, volunteers and family members to all be involved, pull together and give their best as a life comes to an end.

Here are some services that the palliative care team can provide:

Specialist medical care
To become a palliative care physician in Australia and New Zealand, you need to train as a doctor, then specialise in general medicine as a physician, before undergoing further

training to be a registered palliative care physician. It is a big deal to become a palliative care physician in Australia and New Zealand. These are knowledgeable people, so making the most of this knowledge is a 'no brainer'.

Teamwork

Palliative care is a 'team sport'. There are no individual superstars when it comes to good palliative care. From the physician to the registered nurses, social workers, counsellors, carers, volunteers, health advocates and community members, everyone on the team has the same focus: to minimise suffering and treat each life with respect in a holistic manner.

Pain and symptom control

A lot of things go wrong with the functioning of the body as it slows down and prepares for death, and these symptoms can be difficult to manage. Pain is a common symptom in the dying phase of life. The palliative care team know all about the symptoms, what to expect and how to manage them. In addition, the palliative care doctors have access to fantastic pain drugs. If you need a team to make your end of life suffering less, who you gonna call?

End of life planning

Often the palliative care team can help manage and take care of all the medical legal affairs, such as advanced directives and enduring power of attorney. They can help with these documents and paperwork. Their administrative skills are impressive, so ask about and use them.

Terminal care

The last hours of life can be stormy, and syringe drivers are among the inventions that can help make the transition from this life to the next one peaceful and pain free. These devices keep a steady flow of morphine on hand so that there is minimal or no pain suffered in death. The palliative care teams know how to use these devices and how to be kind at the end of life.

There is sometimes a misconception that these devices are used to purposefully end life. This is incorrect, they are used when life is ending, not to end life. This distinction is very important because trust is very important in medical care, and if you don't trust your doctor, either find another doctor or work on your trust issues.

Family focus

The palliative care team not only provides care for the person dying, but for the whole family. They know that dying affects the husbands, wives, children, grandchildren, friends and family too. They have a broad view of care, and they are able to tie the loose ends together.

When it comes to the last days of life or the last months of life, I strongly recommended that you get in touch with a palliative care team. My experience is that these people care for all the right reasons. They are the compassionate ones, and in my mind, the true heroes of medicine.

As with all things there is not always a perfect solution. Some of the conversations are tough and some of the choices are difficult. Palliative care is not about making dying go away, it is about making dying better.

Do not be afraid of the palliative care referral. My best advice is to seek an early palliative care referral when you have an incurable illness. The palliative care journey is gentle and much kinder than the DIY stuff most people try to endure on their own.

If I was going to vote for the best healthcare providers, the palliative care team will always come up tops. Thank you to these selfless people who are prepared to accept dying and to walk in compassion with those who are dying.

Chapter 27

The Unsung Heroes

While the palliative care team may be the medical heroes and, as such, deserving of a medal, none are more deserving than the carers of those who are dying. People don't choose to be carers, caring chooses them. Misfortune happens unexpectedly, and people are thrust into this position without their choice or consent. Often they have few skills in their newfound role. They do their best, and most carers do care most of the time, but there are times when it becomes impossible. There are many things at stake.

Carers suffer all the emotions of the dying. They have the fear, denial, anger, depression, bargaining and guilt that are common in dying. But then there are additional emotions of frustration. Sometimes the only hope seems to be wishing that the person they love and care for will just die! With this comes terrible guilt about being a bad person and being uncaring and unloving. Added to this is exhaustion. I can go home after a hard day's work, but carers are never off duty.

- "Judy, can you please get me a glass of water?"
- "Sam, where are my reading glasses?"
- "I need you to take me to the hospital today."
- "I want you to go and do the banking today."
- "Please help me go to the toilet."
- "I don't want to wear those clothes today."
- "This food tastes terrible."

As carers, it is their duty to help the person who is dying. Every demand is made of them, and it can be 'give, give, give'. There is no rest and there is no reprieve. There is often even no thank you! And if you dare complain as a carer, it is you who is being selfish and inconsiderate. Carers have to endure every whim of the dying, brace for every emotional impact of dying, and be a 24-hour servant, non-stop. It feels that way for many, and it is that way for many.

We need a circuit breaker. Carers are not there to be abused, taken for granted, or expected to do inhuman tasks. There should be some rules to this game.

Rule 1: Accept the mission

Are you willing to be a carer? Many people feel they do not have a choice in this. The role is dropped on them, and they have to hold all the baggage. And the baggage does not always smell that good!

Do you accept this mission? It is easy to say, "I don't have a choice." This may be true, and it often is, but *you* still have to accept the mission.

Until you accept the mission, you will consciously or subconsciously be saying "NO!" And it will always be a resentful uphill battle. It is only when you accept and yield to the role that you can be effective.

The best way I can illustrate this is the example of loading a horse into a horse float. The purpose of the horse float is to transfer the horse from point A to point B.

If the horse refuses to get into the float, the job is so much harder—for the horse and everyone else involved. There is pulling and pushing, swearing and cursing, kicking, snorting and biting—and that's just the spectators. The end result of going from point A to point B does not change, but the effort is exhausting.

It's far easier if the horse trots into the float and, away we go! The job done in a minute. What kind of horse are you?

Rule 2: Be informed

If you are going to be a carer, you need to know what is involved and what the scope of the mission is.

- What is the problem or diagnosis?
- What are the symptoms to be aware of?
- What resources do you need?
- Will you require specialised equipment or house modifications?
- What is the prognosis? Is this expected to be a journey of days, weeks, months, or years?

Knowledge is power. Get good at what you do. Ask questions. Ask the indefensible question when you see the doctor: If this was *your* mother or father, what would you do?

Be proactive. Things won't drop into your lap from the sky. You will need to go out and make things happen.

Rule 3: Get external help

This is often the biggest mistake carers make—the misguided belief that we need to do it on our own. If there is a roadside accident or a bushfire, we all know to dial 000 and get help. The same applies to being a carer. The only difference is the telephone number you need to dial.

Get your GP involved. Ask the palliative care services for their help. Speak to a social worker. Use your community resources to help manage this task. Get your family members involved and make use of friends and neighbours. Often there is more help than you realise. Don't be a martyr.

Rule 4: Set boundaries

Be firm about what is okay and what is not okay. Being the servant and slave to the dying person is not okay. If they can tie their own laces, let them. If they can boil an egg, let them. Don't compensate for their illness by rolling over on daily chores and activities. Don't be a bleeding heart; be a sergeant major—you have a mission, soldier!

It is important to clearly communicate what you are

and are not willing to do. Like all games, there has to be a call made if the ball is on the line. In tennis it is called in, in football it is called out. You get to make your own rules.

Rule 5: Take time out
You need time to rest and recover and be yourself. So, make your time out a priority. Get someone else to look after 'the patient' on a Thursday morning, so that you can go play bridge or golf. Don't feel guilty about this.

Rule 6: Talk about it
Join a chat group or a community group of other carers. Swap plans and strategies. Share secrets and tips that work. Find the community in what you are doing—it helps.

Rule 7: Look after yourself
Most carers forsake personal care. They are exhausted, burnt out, unfit, overweight or underweight people. Get enough sleep, get exercise, go for a walk, eat properly, listen to music, meditate, pray, be kind to yourself and good to yourself. This is not selfish; it is essential if you are going to complete the mission.

Rule 8: Don't crash and burn
Don't be a hero. Don't suffer personal injury. For the most part, this is emotional and psychological injury, especially if the person you are caring for is abusive and there are no escape routes. Please do not be embarrassed to seek the

help of a psychologist, counsellor or spiritual leader.

Talk about how you feel and, if you feel frustrated or 'just want to kill the person you are caring for', realise that these are normal feelings. Let off steam regularly before you crash and burn.

Rule 9: Prepare for the destination

The person you are caring for is going to die. As much as they need to prepare for their eventual death, so too do their carers. Learn to let go. There is a time and season for everything, and when the time comes for death to happen, accept this. Let go. Focus on the good things of life, but don't hold onto them too tightly.

It seems easiest to hold on with both hands, but the reality is that it is easier when you open your hands and let go, trusting in the normality and kindness of death. Believe that it will occur at the right time and hopefully in peace. Prepare for this moment, so that it does not overwhelm you. May the kindness you show be returned to you, but please bear in mind that sometimes you have to be cruel to be kind. You may have to show tough love to get the best out of the person you love.

Chapter 28

Bereavement

Why does it hurt so much when someone dies? Why does it hurt so much to die? We have not addressed this very real issue yet. When we have to say goodbye to the ones we love, the pain is unbearable. Our hearts are broken and there is no salve to heal this hurt. It is because of this pain that we would rather turn away from the topic of death and dying. It is more bearable to continue suffering than to say goodbye.

Those who have experienced bereavement will know the deep, deep pain felt in the heart when someone they love dies. Those who are dying know the pain of bereavement as well. This pain is the price we pay for love. When we understand that our love for another person is a beautiful thing, an eternal force that can never be extinguished, and that we must have loved *so much* to feel so much pain, we can know that we have done well.

To put it into perspective: Did *you* feel any pain when *my* mother died? How could you if you did not know her? If you did not know the person she was, how kind she could be, the sense of fun and humour she possessed, the way she would tease and play tricks on us as kids, and how much she cared for and loved us... How could you feel the loss of all these things if you had not experienced them?

But we loved her for all her faults—warts and all. When she died it was not just her body that died; we missed her whole life—all the love that she had packaged together over the years. This is why people cry and hurt so deeply. The love goes missing—both that given and that received. This is the nature of bereavement, and the prerequisite that it comes with the loss of a relationship based on love.

Grief is the intense sorrow those who are dying feel or that we feel when someone has died. But we don't grieve in this way for all people who die. I do not feel bereft when my patients die. I feel loss, and I empathise with their families, but unless I am close to them, and unless I have loved them, I do not feel the pain of bereavement.

Of the 150,000 people who died today, I may feel regret that their lives have ended, I may feel empathy with their families and the loss they may be enduring, but, unless I have loved them, I don't feel grief. The end of their life does not affect me on a personal level. This may seem shocking, but it illustrates that, in order to grieve, we must have loved. The greater our love, the greater our grief.

From this perspective: Is it a bad thing to have loved? Is it a bad thing to love someone so much that it hurts to consider life without them? No! Even in the pain of bereavement, it is still worth having loved them and I am sure that if you were given the chance again you would love them even more.

Just as we need to accept this price of love—to be heart-broken when life is ending or ends—it is also worth remembering that love never ends. We never stop loving people we have loved. Love continues beyond this life and into eternity, and the love we have for each other endures beyond the grave. If you have a hope that reaches beyond this life into the next, your love will be there waiting. It is not over, ever!

If your heart is breaking at the thought of having to say goodbye, I encourage you to demonstrate your love more, and show the person you love how much you love them. Be kind and considerate while you can. Tell them you love them and write it down. And when the time comes to go, love them. For those who remain: keep on loving—even after those we love are gone. Never stop.

We all demonstrate our love in different ways, depending on our personality, our culture and depending on the day. And, in the same way, we all grieve differently. Some people are demonstrative to the point of needing to be tranquilised; others seem to show no emotion at all. Both equally suffer broken hearts.

For those who are dying, the sadness, pain and loss ends. For those who remain, the pain and the loss continues, but life must go on. Even in the time of being broken-hearted, there are things that must be done. You still have to eat, bathe, dress, go to work and buy groceries. Life has to go on.

In this continuing journey of life, we may fear that our love will diminish, or that we will forget the person we loved so much. The pain gets less over time, it softens from unbearable to a dull ache, and it is eventually not part of every day. It is not a betrayal to accept this. Over time our hearts heal up. We are invited to return to participating in life—to go out and take the risk to keep loving.

Rest assured that, although our recollection may dim and fade over time—the scent of our loved one may diminish, and their life may seem an echo—the love we have for them never fades. It comes with this price tag of pain, but to have loved is better than not to have loved. To have been loved is better than to not have known love.

Do not be afraid to love, do not be afraid of grief. Sometimes grief can be so dark and so overwhelming, that we need to get some help. This is not necessarily help to make the pain go away, but to help refocus and point our lives in a new direction. If we consider those we love and their wishes for us, no one expects their loved ones to keep grieving or wants to hold them captive in a cage of sorrow.

There is a time and a season for all things. There is a time for living, and a time for dying. There is a time for grief, and a time for letting go of grief. If your grief is still dragging you down more than six months after the death of someone you loved, please consider letting go a little. Seek out some help to refocus on the life you still have and how to make it awesome.

Chapter 29

Looking The Other Way & Donuts

We have spent all this time talking about death and how to position ourselves for this future event, but we are still alive! We still have an opportunity to make what is left of our lives count. One of the mistakes we make is assuming that we have forever to do the things we want to do, but in reality, we are only given 24 hours each day, and we have to make the most of it. There is no guarantee that there will be another day.

As much as a terminal diagnosis is devastating news, for some people it is less a disaster than an opportunity. For the first time in their lives, they find their purpose and have a reason to live. They realise that life is indeed a gift and that, although life is ending, it has not ended yet. There are still things to do, places to go and things to experience. They manage to break the mundane cycle of existence and get to smell the roses. And, because life is ending, the scent of the roses is particularly sweet. They are thankful for every opportunity to make the most of life.

On one of my weekend ward rounds, I saw Brian, a patient of a colleague. It was soon obvious that he had a very limited prognosis, with perhaps only weeks to live. In our conversation Brian commented, "I have nothing left to live for." He revealed he was essentially waiting to die. While this may have been relevant for Brian, the question does arise for all of us, "What do we have left to live for?"

This is an important question. 'To live' is the opposite of 'to die'. While we may be fully prepared for death, it does not mean we have to give up and stop living. A friend with Stage 4 incurable breast cancer had a practical approach to her illness. She knew the cancer was there, but she was not going to let it stop her from getting on with life. She was going to keep 'doing life'. If the cancer wanted to, it could come with her, but she was not waiting to ask it for permission.

She was not in denial, she experienced the symptoms associated with her disease, she accepted her diagnosis and her prognosis. But while her illness limited her, it did not stop her. It did not stop her being friendly and showing kindness to those around her. She would get in touch and encourage those around her. She knew that every day was an opportunity to make someone else's day great. That was what she was like.

Wendy was left with horrible scars along the back of her neck and scalp after surgery. She had radiation treatment that left her with permanent bald areas. It was disfiguring but she chose to dress up and look good. She did her hair as best she could, tying it up with a scarf so that no one knew about her illness or battle against cancer. And she got on with what she wanted to do. She had cancer, but she had things to do, so the cancer had to fit in with her plans. She was not in denial but in control of her life, because she accepted the inevitability of death and saw each day as a gift.

To look the other way is not to deny death and what lies ahead, but to look up and away from the pit of despair. It means looking at the things that can be done while there is time. There are endless opportunities. Here are our suggestions:

Do a professional photoshoot

I hate posing for photos. I think it is one of my childhood traumas: having to stand ready for a photo and not knowing how you were supposed to smile. When the film was eventually developed, it was obvious that the family photo was a disaster because that was the moment I looked away.

We all have memories of bad photos, and that is exactly why we need to get a proper photoshoot done with a professional. I once had to do a professional photoshoot for work, and what a surprise it was. The photographer made me feel at ease, he added some powder to my skin and some colour to my face, and away he went taking hundreds of photos. He selected three and I was amazed and delighted at how well they captured my essence! It was money well spent.

You owe it to yourself to do this and leave at least one magnificent photo of yourself for posterity.

Plan a party

Why not take time to celebrate your life? Instead of missing out due to not being able to attend your funeral, have the party brought forward. Make it a big event. Invite friends and family, dress up nicely as you would at a wedding, and make it an opportunity to celebrate life and, if you want, *your* life.

This might be a great time to get that photo done at the same time. You will not regret this.

Do something on your bucket list

The 2007 movie *The Bucket List,* directed by Rob Reiner, and starring Jack Nicholson and Morgan Freeman, tells the story of two men with terminal cancer who set out to enjoy unfulfilled wishes and last adventures before they kick the proverbial bucket. It is a fantastic story and, although it ends with the men dying, it lifts the spirit by saying, "Hey, look here—I lived."

What do you want to do before you die? It might be something adventurous like hot air ballooning, skydiving, or swimming with the whales. It may be doing a pottery course and creating your own super ugly pottery piece. If you have never thought about it, give yourself permission to do one 'wow' thing you never imagined.

Write a journal

You are an encyclopedia of experience and knowledge and, if all else fails, a historical wonder. No one has experienced life like you, nor has anyone seen the world through your eyes. I grew up in a dusty mining town called Orkney, in South Africa. I can recall buying hot chips seasoned with salt and vinegar at a small café next to the Elba movie theatre and watching Terence Hill and Bud Spencer in the *Trinity* movies through the blue haze of cigarette smoke.

I remember the Walldorf Café and drinking strawberry milkshakes with my mum, through paper straws that disintegrated half-way through that pleasure. Across the road was the chemist with one of those fancy water-cooling devices and, as kids, we would sneak in and get a paper cup of ice-cold water for free! These are just some of my memories, but they are *mine*, and perhaps if you grew up in Orkney in the 1970s you would remember the same things.

Everyone's story counts—including yours. So, please consider recording it. It does not have to be a huge task.

Be generous

One of the essential things to do in life is to give. There is a real freedom that comes when you can give without expecting anything in return. If you do expect something in return, such as respect or thanks or recognition or honour, it becomes merely a business transaction. Giving and not expecting anything in return is an expression of love, and we all need to experience this joy in our life.

Many people think of giving in financial terms, but it is far more than this. We can give people time by listening to them. Being friendly is a way of giving, and so are acts of service such as helping to take out the bins. You cannot take anything with you when you are gone, so why not consider being a blessing to someone without them even knowing it. Try it. It is good for you.

Forgive

This is a unique and important way of giving. In life we have all experienced loss at the hand of someone else, but equally, none of us are innocent. We all have a black marks in our books. When life is ending, why not let bygones be bygones, and let past offences go? Why not bury the hatchet and make peace? This starts with forgiveness and letting go.

I know there are some things that have happened in life that are unforgivable. But at the end of life, consider letting these go as well. It is not worth holding on to them into eternity. If there is any chance of being reconciled or seeking forgiveness, make use of this opportunity. It will bring healing.

Have a conversation with God

If you have never had a chat with God, why not start now? It is not that complicated; it simply requires time and preferably a quiet place. Not 'quiet' as in 'silent', but a place where you are not rushing around doing things. When you have time, ask God to help you on your journey. Ask Him to be kind and show compassion to you. Wait. And expect an answer. It will come, not necessarily immediately, but it will come.

Make space for donuts

Do one thing each day that affirms your life and says, "Yay, I am alive!" It may be treating yourself or someone else, listening to your favourite song, eating something delicious every day, or simply taking time for yourself. Whatever it is, make a date with yourself, and be kind to yourself.

Imagine if we never became unwell but that our lives all ended suddenly when our time is up. What would you do differently? What would be different?

The chances are that we would continue doing mundane, routine things like getting up, going to work, coming back from work, eating and sleeping. And then it all starts again, up to the point of BANG! Life's over. For so many of us, life is a bit of a hamster wheel, the same thing over and over. Even though we are alive, we never really get to experience living.

With the knowledge that life is ending and is finite, the things that seemed so important, are perhaps no longer as important. There is a real opportunity to enjoy life. A terminal diagnosis is an invitation to get off the hamster wheel. Working to make profits for the company are no longer the most important things in life. Donuts are!

Just because life is ending does not mean that it has

ended. Whether you have days or weeks or months to live, there is the invitation to live. We can do nothing about death, but we have every opportunity to make the most of life.

Please take time to do the things that matter and make you happy in life. Eat donuts! Drink good wine. Enjoy delicious food. Make every minute count—to the last minute. Plan for it. Take risks, be adventurous, have fun, build memories. I am sure you have a list of suggestions, so please get on with doing those things that matter most and that bring you the greatest happiness.

Chapter 30

Putting It All Together

We have covered a lot of ground. We know a lot more now than we did at the beginning of this journey. By now, we are informed about dying and more comfortable with the concepts of death and dying. This gives us an advantage.

One of the things I like to do at dinner parties is to bring up the topic of death and dying. At first there is stunned silence and shock, but it does not last long. We all have a vested interest in dying. We are all curious about this final frontier, this great next adventure, this impossible task. We all know someone who has died or who has experienced bereavement. The conversation quickly turns to personal experiences of bereavement or anecdotes about loss. In these conversations, I am always amazed by how much people want to contribute. If they are given the opportunity, people *do* want to talk about death and share their experience and concerns.

Generally, people know more about dying than they think. They are more equipped than they believe. But that brings us to a sore point. Even if we knew everything about dying and could do a quiz on it with a perfect score, we all still have the problem of eventually having to personally experience death.

I do not want to die, and I do not want you to die. Is there a way out? There isn't, but there is a way through death. We can do it and we will make it. In so many ways, death is like birth, and we have all experienced birth. None of us thinks back to our birth and says, "Wow, that was terrible!" or "That was fantastic!" We simply do not have a memory of birth at all. Yet at the time of birth, we are powerfully and forcefully ejected from our warm and safe little world *in utero*. We undergo significant crushing trauma as we leave the world we know and enter into the one we know now. At the time of death, it will be the same. We will leave this world that we know and enter into the new world.

If we think about this example of pregnancy, all pregnancies have the same outcome. Apart from some of those who have Caesarean sections, pregnancies typically end with a period of travail and the birth of a child. This process of childbirth is the same, regardless of race, religion, culture, geographical location, wealth or education. Each mum-to-be must go through this process of childbirth, and each baby to be born has to go through the same birth process.

What is different in all pregnancies is the preparation for the baby. Each person prepares for the baby in their own unique way. Each way will be culturally appropriate, and each person has to make do with their resources and budgets and where they live. They have to decide on names. When it comes to preparing the babies' rooms they have to decide on colours. The choice of strollers, nappies and clothes are all individual choices.

In addition, each expectant mum has to contend with the symptoms of pregnancy in her unique way. Some people have access to good medical care, with midwives and obstetricians, and others have to make do with the best advice they can get from their parents and grandparents. Most pregnancies are happy and exciting events, but not all pregnancies are positive experiences. The journey to the labour ward is as unique as each person's fingerprints.

When it comes to dying, the same applies. Although we have death in common, we all have our own unique life experience. Our friends and family are unique to us, just as our financial, geographical, cultural, social and religious experiences are also. No one can tell us how to prepare for death. This is our choice! We get to prepare for this time in our lives on our terms. We get to do the best with what we have so that we can meet with death on our own terms.

I hope that the information presented here will make a difference in the way each person prepares for death. Each one will do it in their own unique way.

May our preparation for death be a good one. May there be adventure along the way and may there be good memories. May our wrongs be forgiven and may there be peace in our hearts. May we celebrate and enjoy the life that we have lived and, if we have taken a wrong turn, may we find our way back to the light. May we enjoy ice cream, and the sound of music, and be surrounded by laughter. May we love and be loved and know that we are all valuable.

May you be equipped and ready to face death when it arrives, even if it arrives early. May you leave some of yourself behind so that the world can be richer. May your journey towards the end of life be blessed and safe in God's hands.

I wish you well. I hope that you find time to enjoy the donuts.

Chapter 31

Dying To Understand

We do not know a lot when it comes to dying. As doctors, we can only guess what people feel and think when their life is ending. Knowing this, I realise that this book may be a total failure in terms of addressing the *real* needs of those who are dying. When it comes to dying, I often feel that I may boldly be declaring that the Earth is flat. But, while we may be forgiven for any ignorance, we should not be allowed to get away with remaining ignorant.

How do we not remain ignorant? It is through asking questions. To facilitate death education, we established Dying to Understand, a registered charity to promote death education.

The first purpose of Dying to Understand is to ask for your opinion and insight, to ask questions and to talk about dying so that we become less ignorant. This sharing of knowledge is the starting point of our journey to be good at death education.

Our second purpose is to provide a point of contact for all those who are struggling on this journey. We are always available at admin@dyingtounderstand.com and if you need to reach out and get in touch, please do. Perhaps you have a question, comment, a point of improvement or some criticism, or genuine praise for what we are trying to do. Regardless, please get in touch. We would love to hear from you.

The third purpose of Dying to Understand is to build and develop resources for those on this journey.

The final purpose of our charity is to encourage and fund research. We support projects that make life better where there is suffering. Funding will enable us to have a free hand to grow our resources. If you are able to contribute, we will be most grateful.

We know that we are moving out of the darkness into the light. We hope that what we previously knew will become obsolete as our knowledge and understanding grows. We know that we are better than we were, but not as great as we can be. We invite you to become part of this journey by sharing your story with us.

Please support our charity by visiting: dyingtounderstand.com.

Epilogue

My motivation for writing this book has been to offer hope. For me the greatest hope is that of my faith. I believe that when I die I will I be going to heaven and be reunited with God. I believe that this will be a homecoming, a celebration and a time of great joy despite the sorrows associated with dying.

How can this be possible? Well, through faith. We touched on spirituality and the invisible and intangible nature of spirituality. If it makes no sense, it requires that leap of faith. It requires a willingness to let go and trust God. If you were on the top storey of a burning building and were required to jump through the dark smoke into the safe hands of the firemen below, would you be able to do it on hearsay alone? It will depend on your trust in the firemen. It will depend on your respect for the flames. The same applies to an experience with God. Is there a God you can trust with your life?

I grew up in a Christian home and in a Christian culture, with a Christian religion. It had no real meaning to me, and it was a chore. This is the nature of religion; it is a chore, something that must be done or obeyed—or else. I was not convinced. If you are religious and it is not offering you any joy or if you are wary of religion, join the club.

In April 1980 on a swimming tour, while we were staying at Midmar Dam in Natal, I reluctantly and out of Christian duty, agreed to attend an early morning prayer meeting with some of the Christian kids on the tour. At 6 am in the morning, the sun was just breaking over the water when I had an encounter with Jesus. It was a simple encounter and an easy conversation. It was both an invitation and an *instruction*.

"Come and follow me."

I said, "Yes."

In that encounter, something in me was transformed; something that was dead in me came to life; something that was broken in me was restored. I experienced joy and peace. I was made alive. I knew Jesus in person. It was no longer a religious experience but a personal experience. Based on this transformational experience, I am happy to follow Jesus, and I can recommend Him to you.

I believe that everyone can have the same experience. It is not based on merit. It is based on trust in Him. Can you make the commitment when He calls you to follow Him? Dare you ask Him to help you or do you trust someone else? You have absolutely nothing to lose by turning to Him for help.

You are also invited to follow Jesus. He may take you

where you do not want to go, but follow Him. He may take you where you never thought it is possible to go, but follow Him. He may take you through the fire, but follow Him. He is so worth following.

Get hold of a Bible and read it. Not as an instruction manual, but a love letter. Hidden in its pages are life and wisdom and truth. Speak to Jesus, say this simple prayer if you do not know where to start:

"Lord Jesus, help me."

If you need more information, please contact me at admin@dyingtounderstand.com and I will be in touch.

For now, I wish you well and Godspeed. I hope to see you on the other side.

About the Author

Colin grew up in the mining town of Orkney in South Africa. He completed his schooling at St Stithians College in Johannesburg and started his medical training at the University of Pretoria. As a young man, Colin had an extraordinary number of encounters with death. He witnessed his first death in his teens while at the local swimming pool, where a young man fell off an unprotected grandstand and died instantly. Following this experience, and by the age of 24, Colin was witness to three separate motor vehicle deaths and a death at a wedding. He was also exposed to death as a medical student. Death was a topic that Colin could not avoid.

After completing his medical training and compulsory military training, Colin and his wife Mathilde spent a year in Hull, UK. After this experience in the oncology department, Colin returned to South Africa to specialise. He completed his training as a radiation oncologist in 1998 and shortly after that moved to New Zealand for a two-year adventure. Colin completed a Diploma of Palliative Medicine while in New Zealand, and his two-year adventure turned out to be a fantastic five-year experience. Colin and his family returned to South Africa in 2003.

As an oncologist, Colin became aware of the lack of conversation around death and dying and this led him to write his first book *About dying: How to live in the face of death*. It was well received, but it lacked what Colin viewed as substance. Following his research project on death education, and with a colleague and a friend both facing terminal illness, Colin started writing on death, using the writing to express his views about the dying process. His friend and colleague never got to read the book, but Colin hopes there may be others who get to read this book and that it will make a difference in the way they live their life and complete their life.

Colin continues to work on the Sunshine Coast as a radiation oncologist. He is also the founder of Dying to Understand, a charity promoting death education. He can be reached via the charity at admin@dyingtounderstand.com.

Outside of work, Colin has a 'full-time job' as a husband to his beautiful wife Mathilde, a father to four fantastic adult children, and a labourer on his acreage on the Sunshine Coast.

www.ingramcontent.com/pod-product-compliance
Lightning Source LLC
Chambersburg PA
CBHW050307010526
44107CB00055B/2142